KETO DIET

COOKBOOK AFTER 50

HOW TO START A KETO DIET AFTER FIFTY. 250 EASY LOW-CARB RECIPES AND A 30 DAYS MEAL PLAN TO LOSE WEIGHT NATURALLY AND HEALTHILY AND FEEL YOUNGER.

ELIZABETH VOGEL

TABLE OF CONTENTS

Introduction

Keto diet has become the traditional craze that has captivated our attention. In this context, I will be explaining the details about the diet, including the benefits and the foods that should be consumed while following it.

What Is Keto Diet and Who Is it for?

This is considered as a diet that is low in carbohydrate content and is essentially high in fat content. It is similar to the other low carbohydrate diets in several ways, but there are several points of differences as well.

As you consume a diet that has low carb content, you must fill up that loss with moderate amounts of protein that may also include an increased intake of fat. As your carbohydrate intake decreases, while you follow this diet, your body goes into a state which is defined as ketosis, where the quantity of fat that you have been consuming from your diet is specifically used by the system to flame the fat to provide you with the energy.

Meaning of the Word 'Keto'

This diet has been given such a name because it induces your body to burn the fat that results in the formation of small molecules of fuel known as 'ketones.' Your body uses this source of fuel as an alternative for glucose (blood sugar) when the glucose quantity is in shortage.

While you are consuming a relatively low number of calories or carb, it is your liver that is producing ketone molecules from the fat content. These ketones are then serving as the fuel source all over the body and especially to the brain. Most of the energy that our body produces by burning fat or glucose is utilized by the brain, which is considered as the hungry organ of the human system. And, when we are on a keto diet, we usually lower the carb content and increase the fat content; therefore, the amount of fat that we consume cannot be directly utilized by the brain. It can only run on ketones or glucose.

The body switches the entire supply of fuel to run on ketones produced from fat when we are on such a diet, and hence it burns fat for 24-7. The level of insulin drops because of low-calorie intake, and this causes the burning of fat to increase dramatically as accessing the fat stores becomes easier.

Besides helping to lose weight, there are several other health benefits, which include making you feel less hungry, and the energy is also supplied steadily by burning the fat without the formation of peaks and valleys of sugar that occurs when high-carb meals are consumed. This may also aid you to remain alert and stay focused.

This is also the way by which you can skip the habit of fasting. Nobody can fast consistently. But staying on a low carb diet is. It results in ketosis where you get the power of eating indefinitely and still getting the energy required by your body without having to fear for increasing the blood sugar level.

Who Is This Diet Not for?

If we are keeping the controversies related to following a ketogenic diet aside, it appears to be safe for most of the people. Then come the three groups of people who require to consider this diet, especially:

- A person who takes medication for diabetes, for example, insulin

- A person who is under medication for having high blood pressure

- If a mother breastfeeds

There are also other people, especially adults, who have health issues, for example, obesity can have lots of benefits for the ketogenic diet. Only if you are under medication, you need to consult your physician before following this diet.

What Are the Benefits of the Keto Diet?

This diet has been facing many controversies since it was introduced. Some people believe that switching to this diet can cause heart-related problems because of the high amount of fat that is consumed and increases the level of cholesterol too. But this diet has proved its worth as beneficial and healthy by several scientific studies that have been conducted to test its effect on the human body.

Here are the eight health benefits of consuming a low-carb and ketogenic diet that has been proven by scientists.

Reduces Appetite

The biggest problem faced by people who want to lose their weight is the feeling of hunger. Feeling hungry is intended as the worst part about dieting. This is the primary reason behind people surrendering to the concept of dieting.

However, a diet that includes low carbohydrate intake automatically reduces the appetite. Cutting the carbs and filling up space with increased consumption of protein and fat has been proved by researchers to be the easiest way of eating fewer calories.

Abdominal Cavity Loses the Maximum Fat

Various types of fat are present in different body parts. The places that store fat determines the way it affects health and how it risks diseases.

Many researchers have shown that overweight men are typically so because of the high accumulation of two fat types- visceral fat in the cavity of the abdomen and the subcutaneous fat present beneath the skin. A rise in the amount of visceral fat leads to insulin resistance and inflammation, which tends to push the metabolic dysfunction.

But people who are on this keto diet has shown to reduce these fat stored mainly in the abdominal cavity drastically. And this reduction, with time, should lead to a reduction in type II diabetes and other heart diseases.

Increase in Levels of Cholesterol

HDL, which is the short form for high-density lipoprotein, is often considered as the 'good' type of cholesterol in human beings. People who have a low density of lipoprotein are at a greater risk of facing heart problems.

The best way to increase HDL cholesterol is by including more fat in the diet, which can be done by following the keto diet.

High Blood Pressure May Drop

Most of the diseases, for example, kidney failure, strokes, and heart diseases, are triggered by an increase in blood pressure. This is considered as a significant chance factor in many people. Switching to a diet that decreases the carbohydrate content can be an effective way to decrease the hazards of such diseases, which may ultimately help you to live longer.

Remedial for Various Brain Morbidities

Your brain is the only organ that needs to be fed constantly. This also the organ that requires glucose as the source of energy, as there are parts that can only burn this sugar. This is the reason behind the production of glucose by burning protein when we consume fewer carbohydrates.

Yet, there are parts in your brain that can burn ketones too. This is the mechanism that has been made to use for decades for treating children with epilepsy who does not respond to medicines.

Compelling against Metabolic Syndrome

This syndrome is highly related to the risk of heart diseases and diabetes. Precisely, this syndrome is an assemblage of various disorders such as:

Abdominal obesity

Low levels of good cholesterol (HDL)

Increased levels of fasting blood sugar

Elevated blood sugar

High triglycerides

However, all these symptoms can be effectively treated by following a diet low in the carb content. These conditions eventually get eliminated by following such a diet.

Reduced Insulin and Blood Sugar Levels

Diabetes resistance to insulin is a problem that is faced by people across the world. For such people, a diet that has a low content of carbohydrates can be particularly effective.

When people who have diabetes were asked to start such a diet, it was seen that this reduced the dose of insulin by almost fifty-five percent. In a study conducted with people who have type II diabetes, it was seen that they had reduced the intake of medicines by ninety-five percent. Thus following such a diet has been proved to lower blood sugar and insulin effectively.

Weight Loss

The simplest way known as far for losing weight is by cutting out those carbohydrate-containing foods from your diet. This is considered because lowering the carbohydrates consumption helps your body to get rid of the excess water, lower the levels of insulin that lead to rapid weight loss in the first week of following this diet. This is an effective way by which people lose weight significantly by restricting their carb consumption without being hungry.

Foods to Eat on Keto Diet

This diet is gaining popularity recently. This diet is believed to be very effective against diabetes, weight loss, and epilepsy. Other pieces of evidence show this diet to be helpful for the therapy of certain cancers and other diseases like Alzheimer's disease. The carbohydrate in this diet is limited to twenty to fifty grams each day. Although it looks like a challenge still this can be achieved by including several nutritious foods in the diet.

Here is the list of some foods that can be beneficial as well as lip-smacking for those finding it hard to cut the carb out of their diet.

Seafood

Shellfishes are foods that are known to be very keto-friendly. Salmons are highly nutritious and are loaded with potassium, selenium, and vitamin B yet free from carbohydrates. Shrimps and crabs also contain no carb in them. Omega-3 fats are present in high amounts in sardines, salmons, and mackerel, which are highly beneficial for lowering the insulin level and increasing its sensitivity in obese people.

Avocado

This fruit is considered to be incredibly nutritious. They have essential fibers, which form seven out of nine parts of the carbs, so the net carb content is only two grams. Potassium is the most important mineral that can make it easy to get used to a ketogenic diet.

Moreover, this fruit can help by improving the levels of triglyceride and cholesterol.

Vegetables

The carbohydrate content and calories are extremely low in non-starchy veggies but have handsome amounts of other nutrients and minerals. They have certain fibers that are not easily digested like other carbohydrates. Fruits like beets, yams or potatoes are enough to put you over the total limit of carbohydrate for the whole day. Vegetables like cauliflower, broccoli, and kale have been connected to reduced risks of cancer. Besides, these fruits and veggies also contain vitamin C and antioxidants.

Poultry and Meat

They are an essential source of protein that helps in maintaining muscle mass even when you are down on carbohydrates. These foods are zero in carbohydrate and high vitamin B content and other minerals like zinc, selenium, and potassium.

Coconut and Olive Oil

Coconut is a well-suited fruit for this diet. They have medium-chain triglycerides that are completely different from the long-chain fats, which are used as the swift supply of energy. People who are suffering from disorders of the nervous system and brain are, in fact, given coconut to increase their levels of the ketone. A mixture of lauric acid found in coconut with the triglycerides is known to keep the ketosis levels sustained.

Oleic acid present in olive oil reduces heart risks. Moreover, phenol is present in this oil (extra virgin) that decreases inflammation and improves the function of the artery.

Nuts and Seeds

Nuts have high amounts of fat and fiber, which can help you to feel fuller and thus reduce the calorie intake. They have very low carbohydrate content, which makes them ideal to be included in such a diet.

CHAPTER 1:

What Is A Keto Diet?

As I already mentioned, the ketogenic diet is a perfect combination of an equal number of macros essential for the perfect and healthy functioning of the human body.

This diet is mostly focused on foods that are rich in fats, while carbohydrates are considerably lowered.

If you hadn't heard about the keto diet, you probably did not know that eating meals without balanced (or reduced) macros (carbohydrates, proteins, fats, and fibers) will lead to weight and fat.

When you provide your body with foods containing large amounts of carbohydrates (and fats and protein), your body stimulates insulin development, leading to leptin resistance. Slowly but surely, your body weight will increase. Not every organism is the same, but providing the body with unhealthy amounts of carbs combined with fats and proteins (without any physical activity) is a surefire way to end up obese.

How was the ketogenic diet discovered?

Although this diet may have only recently become popular, it is not new at all. It is almost a century old.

In the early 1920s, Johns Hopkins Medical Center researchers had a mission to find a way to decrease the number of seizures in epileptic children. It seemed like an impossible mission to help epileptic children. Still, after thorough research, the researchers discovered that food rich in carbohydrates is the main reason epileptic children have frequent seizures.

They decided to start a new diet and observe the results. The epileptic patients started following the ketogenic diet, which consisted of foods rich in fats and proteins. With only a small amount of carbohydrates, it was discovered that this diet significantly decreased the seizures.

However, as in everything, there were exceptions. The keto diet did not work for everyone; about 30 percent of epileptic children did not react to this diet. Naturally, the epileptic children still had to be observed and take their medications, but the low-carb diet turned out to be quite a relief for most of them.

Before this research, some form of the keto diet had existed, even in ancient Greece and India. Fasting and reducing the consumption of foods with carbs was nothing new to these people.

Historians have found ancient writings that carefully explained how a diet helps in managing epileptic seizures. In ancient times, people were giving up foods for a day or two and were facing complete relief (especially people with epilepsy).

Because fasting can be quite a challenge, over time, the keto diet took on the form it has today. You get to eat enough, and you cut out only carbohydrates (or eat them in reduced amounts).

Before the Johns Hopkins Medical Center research, French doctors discovered a way to reduce epileptic seizures with suitable foods. At the beginning of the twentieth century in France, an experiment was conducted in which about 20 patients with epilepsy followed a new diet (mostly vegetarian) that was low in carbs. By then, the doctors were using potassium bromide to treat the patients, but it turned out that this did not work well in terms of their mental abilities. This early form of keto was combined with intermittent fasting and showed good results. About ten percent of the treated patients reacted positively to the new way of eating. Also, they were in a good mental state and did not need to take potassium bromide.

Slowly but surely, the ketogenic diet found its way to people without epilepsy. It was one of the diets that helped people stay full and healthy and lose weight fast.

How Keto Works
We will focus on how this diet works and how your body transitions from one way of functioning to another.

As mentioned before, the ketogenic diet was used mainly to lower the incidence of seizures in epileptic children.

People wanted to check out how the keto diet would work with an entirely healthy person as things usually go.

This diet makes the body burn fats much faster than it does carbohydrates. The carbohydrates that we take in through food are turned into glucose, one of the leading "brain foods." So, once you start following the keto diet, food with reduced carbohydrates is forcing the liver to turn all the fats into fatty acids and ketone bodies. The ketones go to the brain and take the place of glucose, becoming the primary energy source. This is how your body turns towards the next best energy source to function correctly.

This diet's primary purpose is to make your body switch from the way it used to function to an entirely new way of creating energy, keeping you healthy and alive.

Once you start following the ketogenic diet, you will notice that things are changing, first and foremost, in your mind. Before, carbohydrates were your main body 'fuel' and were used to create glucose so that your brain could function. Now you no longer feed yourself with them.

In the beginning, most people feel odd because their natural food is off the table. When your menu consists of more fats and proteins, it is natural to feel that something is missing.

Your brain alarms you that you haven't eaten enough and sends you signals that you are hungry. It is literally "panicking" and telling you that you are starving, which is not correct. You get to eat, and you get to eat plenty of good food, but not carbs.

This condition usually arises during the first day or two. Afterward, people get used to their new eating habits.

Once the brain "realizes" that carbs are no longer an option, it will focus on "finding" another abundant energy source: in this case, fats.

Not only is your food rich in fats, but your body contains stored fats in large amounts. As you consume more fats and fewer carbs, your body "runs" on the fats, both consumed and stored. The best thing is that, as the fats are used for energy, they are burned. This is how you get a double gain from this diet.

Usually, it will take a few days of consuming low-carb meals before you start seeing visible weight loss results. You will not even have to check your weight because the fat layers will be visibly reduced.

This diet requires you to lower your daily consumption of carbs to only 20 grams. For most people, this transition from a regular carb-rich diet can be quite a challenge. Most people are used to eating bread, pasta, rice, dairy products, sweets, soda, alcohol, and fruits, so quitting all these foods might be challenging.

However, this is all in your head. If you manage to win the "battle" with your mind and endure the diet for a few days, you will see that you no longer have cravings as time goes by. Plus, the weight loss and the fat burn will be a great motivation to continue with this diet.

The keto diet practically makes the body burn fats much faster than carbohydrates; the foods you consume with this diet are quite rich in fats. Carbs will be there, too, but at far lower levels than before. Foods rich in carbohydrates are the body's primary fuel or the brain's food. (Our bodies turn carbs into glucose.) Because there are hardly any carbohydrates in this diet, the body will have to find a substitute source of energy to keep itself alive.

Many people who don't truly need to lose weight and are completely healthy still choose to follow the keto diet because it is a great way to keep their meals balanced. Also, it is the perfect way to cleanse the body of toxins, processed foods, sugars, and unnecessary carbs. The combination of these things is usually the main reason for heart failure, some cancers, diabetes, cholesterol, or obesity.

If you ask a nutritionist about this diet, they will recommend it without a doubt. So, if you feel like cleansing your body and starting a diet that will keep you healthy, well-fed, and slender, perhaps the keto diet should be your primary choice.

And what is the best thing about it (besides the fact that you will balance your weight and lower the risk of many diseases)?

There is no yo-yo effect. The keto diet can be followed forever and has no side effects. It does not restrict you from following it for a few weeks or a month. Once you get your body to keto foods, you will not think about going back to the old ways of eating your meals.

CHAPTER 2:

Know And Calculate Your Macros

Macros

As stated above, macronutrients are an essential part of your everyday life. These nutrients are what give you energy and allow your metabolism to function properly. Without the right number of certain macros, you will find you probably have trouble losing weight. Macronutrients all have a caloric value, but rather than just tracking calories, you track the nutrients that make up those calories. This ensures you have the right ones for your body structure, because if you don't have the correct types of calories, you may not be giving your body the proper nutrition it needs to function at its best. Everyone's body is different, so they have to track their macros differently. This is why calorie counting diets never work. You can't just eat anything that falls within your calorie limit, because you may be getting too much of one macronutrient, but not enough of the others.

Macros are broken down into three categories. These categories are as follows:

Fat

Yes, fat is a necessary part of a normal diet. There are actual fats that are good for you and essential for a healthy diet. You do not want to shy away from consuming these as your metabolism will not be able to function, because this\ is the driving force behind a well-tuned body. Fat is used and turned into energy. This energy is used to regulate your hormones, form cell membranes, and improve brain function. These fats also help to give you healthy skin, hair, and nails. They aid in the regulation of temperature and carry vitamins throughout your body as well. There are four types of fats:

Monounsaturated Fat: These facts are good for your heart, and help decrease the level of unhealthy fat in your bloodstream. There are several foods that you can eat that contain a healthy amount of these fats. These include avocados, olive oil, peanut butter, and almonds.

Polyunsaturated Fat: These facts are necessary for healthy brain function, skin and hair growth, prevention of heart attacks, and control of blood pressure and clotting. There are two categories of polyunsaturated fats – linoleic (omega-6) and linolenic (omega-3). These essential fats cannot be produced from other fats in your body and must be obtained through your diet. You can find them in foods like salmon, tuna, nuts, seeds, and soybean oil.

Saturated Fat: These facts are also known as animal fats because they are contained in many types of meat and dairy products, such as milk, cheese, butter, and cream. Consumption of these fats in your diet should be limited. Too much can raise your cholesterol and cause negative health implications for your heart and blood pressure.

Trans Fat: These are the unhealthiest of fats, and should only be consumed in minute doses. These fats severely increase levels of bad cholesterol and can lead to the clogging of your arteries. They are found in many processed foods such as margarine, deep-fried take-outs, and baked goods like biscuits, cakes, and pastries.

Those are the four types of fats and how they affect you. Remember, unsaturated fats are best, and trans fats are the worst. If you monitor your fat intake well, you should be able to maintain maximum health.

Carbohydrates

Contrary to many misleading diet claims, carbs are not the enemy. They are an important component of your everyday diet. These are broken down into energy used to digest food, and also create enzymes in the small intestine that allow you to pass out all waste without getting ill. Carbohydrates comprise of five forms:

Monosaccharides: These simple sugars form the most basic units of underlined carbohydrates. They are also known as glucose or fructose and are found in many natural foods, such as berries, honey, and syrups or nectars. Monosaccharides are a water-soluble sugar that sweetens these foods naturally and gives them a golden brown color when reduced.

Disaccharides are also known as sucrose, a substance that acts as a natural sweetener in foods. It can be in crystal or liquid form and is found in many natural foods. Lactose, found in milk, is also considered to be a disaccharide. Lactose is what gives milk its sweet taste, and can be an allergen for some individuals.

Oligosaccharides: Do not occur very frequently in foods. This form of carbohydrate serves as added fiber and has a probiotic function. Found in foods such as onions, lentils, and beans, they contain the enzymes that convert into fecal matter through the waste process.

Polysaccharides: Or starches, are the most abundant of carbohydrates that are out there. Many people associate carbs with starchy foods, rather than veggies and fruits. You have been told that these foods are bad, but that is quite the opposite. Starches are one of the most important components of your diet as they help to absorb nutrients into the bloodstream. Polysaccharides are contained in foods such as wheat, oats, rye, barley, potatoes, and legumes.

Protein

This forms one of the essential elements of our diet, as it builds muscle and allows it to heal after an injury. It also contains a lot of iron, which helps regulate your blood composition, and prevents you from becoming anemic.

Protein is formed from a combination of twenty amino acids. There are nine essential amino acids (cannot be made by the body and must be sourced through your diet) and eleven non-essential amino acids that your body can produce. All of these acids are necessary to thrive, but the amount they need to be present varies. Protein allows you to have a strong and healthy body, which is the goal of any diet. Being healthy will allow you to live life to the fullest, without always being sluggish and tired. Essential amino acids are in foods such as eggs, animal proteins, quinoa, soy, and kidney beans. Supplementation of non-essential amino acids in the body can be done by consuming whole foods like nuts, grains, meats, fruits, and vegetables.

Macronutrients Breakdown

Most dieticians say you should have a 40/30/30 diet when breaking down macros. This means forty percent protein, thirty percent fat, and thirty percent carbs. However, this concept has been superseded by the block diet theory (e.g., Zone and Paleo). This approach extols that individuals require more carbohydrates than protein. This has been the style that athletes adhere to religiously as it is seen to produce the best results.

The framework for this breakdown is for every pound you weigh, and you need between 0.5 and 1 gram of protein depending on your activity level. And for every seven grams of protein you require, you need nine grams of carbs and three grams of fats.

Tracking

You can track your macros by looking up the nutritional information online and then noting them down. This is the way a lot of old-school athletes do it. However, you can also use a handy phone app or go online to resources such as MyFitnessPal, a website that will help you track your macros and even look up nutritional info for you.

Why You Should Track

You should track what you eat, that way you can be sure that you are meeting your nutritional requirements. For those with busy lifestyles, it helps to time when you last date to ensure your mealtimes are balanced. This will serve to call out instances of late-night binging and promote a habit of regular eating for optimum body metabolism. Get a little planner, use it to write down what you consume each day, and keep track of its macronutrient value.

Tracking the types of foods you consume will also enable you to see the progress you have made in cleaning up your diet, as well as how you have improved in splitting your macros up evenly without going over or under. The more validation you have of your progress, the more you will want to align with the flexible dieting methodology for ultimate success.

The main advantage of tracking your macros, specifically, is that you can optimize the ratios for your specific body needs. For example, if you are doing high-intensity exercise and weight training, you can maximize results by increasing your carbohydrate intake. Your body may also respond better by slightly reducing your fat intake to compensate for the added carbs, leading to better performance and muscle definition.

Remember, each person has a different baseline of metabolism and body function. It may take a month or so of tweaking your ratios to find what works optimally for your specific bodily needs.

Why Do I Track with 100% Accuracy?

Unless you are a hard-core bodybuilder, tracking with is not a requirement. Flexible dieting allows you to consume foods. For example, to reach 300g carb, then anything from 290 to 310 grams is fine. The net difference in calories is negligible and will not negatively impact your diet results. Often the breakdown of restaurant foods and take-outs may be slightly off, so this buffer provides relief from the over-analysis of each meal.

Conversely, you should take slightly more caution when consuming fats as they contain double the calories of protein and carbs. If you aim to eat only 50 grams of fat a day, then 45 to 55 grams will be okay. That being said, do not stress over exact macros, just try to come within a small deviation of your target. Your body does not detect perfect macros, so there is no point in getting them right. Stressing out about eating perfectly can be counterproductive to your physique goals, so don't freak out if you miss your macros now and then!

Should I Compensate For Remaining Calories?

Once you have hit your macros split for the day, people often find that they have not met their calculated calorie intake. Don't worry too much about this, as it is a common occurrence when undertaking flexible dieting. Over time, the diversity of food options that you consume tends to balance out any caloric deficits. In practice, this means that today's slight deficit will compensate for tomorrow's slight excess. Trying to fill in the remaining calories will throw off your macros split for the day and make the diet much more difficult to practice. Focus on achieving your ratio, and the rest will even out during the week.

CHAPTER 3:

Breakfast Recipes

Peanut Butter Chocolate Protein Shake

Preparation Time: 2 minutes

Cooking Time: 0 minute

Serving: 1

Ingredients:

1 cup whole milk or unsweetened plant-based milk - 1 cup of ice cubes

Two tablespoons natural peanut butter - One scoop chocolate protein powder

Directions:

Put the milk, ice, peanut butter, and protein powder in a blender and blend until smooth, scraping down the sides as needed.

Try to choose a protein powder with 20 to 30 grams of protein per serving and no added sugar. Most are sweetened with stevia or another non-nutritive sweetener. My favorite protein powder is the Garden of Life Sport Organic Plant-Based Protein, chocolate flavor.

Protein shakes are a perennial favorite because they're easy to make and even easier to enjoy. I make a version of this shake nearly every day and appreciate the way it keeps me feeling full and energized until lunchtime.

Nutrition:

Calories: 389 - Fat: 25g - Saturated Fat9g

Sodium: 325mg - Total Carbohydrates19g - Net Carbohydrates: 17g

Fiber: 2g - Sugar: 17g - Protein: 26g

Creamy Dreamy Green Smoothie

Preparation Time: 2 minutes

Cooking Time: 0 minute

Serving: 1

Ingredients:

One small avocado, pitted, peeled, and diced

One lime, peeled

1 cup spinach

1 cup unsweetened almond milk

1 cup of ice cubes

One tablespoon almond butter

2 or 3 drops liquid stevia

Directions:

Put the avocado, lime, spinach, almond milk, ice, almond butter, and liquid stevia in a blender and blend until smooth, scraping down the sides as needed.

To keep avocados fresher longer, cut them in half, remove the pit, and scoop out the flesh. Cut it into pieces, place on a parchment-lined baking sheet, and freeze until solid.

The antioxidants, vitamins, and minerals in this smoothie make a healthy way to start your day. Antioxidants are found primarily in plants, and they combat oxidative stress in your body (think of it like rust forming on a car), thereby helping to keep you looking and feeling your best.

Nutrition:

Calories: 454 - Fat: 39g

Saturated Fat: 5g - Sodium: 220mg

Total Carbohydrates: 28g - Net Carbohydrates: 11g

Fiber: 17g - Sugar: 3g

Protein: 9g

Blueberry-Flax Yogurt Parfait

Preparation Time: : 5 minutes

Cooking Time: 0 minute

Serving: 1

Ingredients:

½ cup whole-milk plain yogurt

One tablespoon ground flax meal

2 to 3 teaspoons liquid stevia

One teaspoon extra-virgin olive oil

¼ teaspoon lemon zest

2 or 3 drops freshly squeezed lemon juice

¼ cup fresh blueberries

Two tablespoons chopped toasted pecans

Direction:

Put the yogurt in a small bowl.

Stir in the flax meal, liquid stevia, olive oil, lemon zest, and lemon juice.

Top with the blueberries and pecans.

To make this plant-based, choose plain cashew- or coconut-based yogurt. My favorite is the full-fat variety of Forager.

The probiotics in yogurt—whether dairy yogurt or a plant-based variety—add to the good bacteria in your gut. This improves digestion, aids in weight loss, increase energy, and even brightens your mood. That's a lot for some teeny little bacteria!

Nutrition:

Calories: 367 - Fat: 31g - Saturated Fat: 5g

Sodium: 58mg - Total Carbohydrates: 22g - Net Carbohydrates: 10g

Fiber: 12g - Sugar: 6g - Protein: 13g

Salted Peanut Butter and Chocolate Yogurt Cup

Preparation Time: : 5 minutes

Cooking Time: 0 minute

Serving: 1

Ingredients:

½ cup whole-milk plain yogurt

2 or 3 drops liquid stevia

Two tablespoons creamy natural peanut butter

One tablespoon no-sugar-added chocolate chips

Pinch flaky sea salt

Directions:

One tablespoon coarsely chopped salted peanuts

Put the yogurt in a small bowl.

Stir in the liquid stevia.

Add the peanut butter and chocolate chips, and stir until partly combined.

Top with the salt and peanuts.

Can you tell I love the combination of peanut butter and chocolate? I make no apologies—when you're transitioning to a low-carb diet, delicious and familiar flavor combinations make it much easier to stick with the plan.

This works equally well with other nut kinds of butter, such as hazelnut or almond butter.

Nutrition:

Calories: 315 - Fat: 25g - Saturated Fat: 7g

Sodium: 439mg - Total Carbohydrates: 18g - Net Carbohydrates: 15g

Fiber: 3g - Sugar: 9g - Protein: 15g

Crunchy Nut and Seed Granola

Preparation Time: : 5 minutes

Cooking Time25 minutes

Serving: Makes 6 cups (12½-cup servings)

Ingredients:

1 cup raw unsalted pecans

1 cup raw unsalted almonds

1 cup raw unsalted sunflower seeds

2 cups unsweetened coconut flakes

1 cup raw unsalted pepitas

¼ cup sesame seeds

Two teaspoons ground cinnamon

½ cup of coconut oil

½ cup unsweetened applesauce

One teaspoon pure vanilla extract

5 or 6 drops liquid stevia

Directions:

Put the pecans, almonds, and sunflower seeds in a food processor and pulse until coarsely ground.

Add the coconut flakes, pepitas, sesame seeds, and cinnamon, and pulse once or twice, or until just combined.

In a medium bowl, whisk the coconut oil, applesauce, vanilla, and liquid stevia, then pour into the food processor and pulse once or twice again until just combined.

Spread the mixture onto the baking sheet, transfer to the oven, and bake for 10 minutes.

Stir, then return the baking sheet to the oven and bake for another 10 minutes.

Stir, then flatten with the back of a spatula, as if you're making dessert bars—Bake for a final 5 minutes, or until the mixture is golden brown and somewhat dried out.

Most granola recipes are loaded with sugar; if you look at the nutrition facts, you might mistake some for dessert! This version is built around filling protein and healthy fats, with a hint of sweetness from stevia. It includes pepitas (shelled pumpkin seeds), too. Don't fear the applesauce in this recipe! It adds only 1 gram of carbohydrate per serving and brings a nice bit of sweet and tart to the granola. Serve this over yogurt or with a splash of milk and a handful of berries for a delicious low-carb breakfast.

Allow the mixture to cool completely before storing. This will help the granola form crisp chunks. Store for up to one month in an airtight container.

Nutrition:

Calories: 399;

Fat: 38g;

Saturated Fat: 18g;

Sodium: 9mg;

Total Carbohydrates: 11g;

Net Carbohydrates: 5g;

Fiber: 6g;

Sugar: 3g;

Protein: 8g

Classic Pancakes

Preparation Time: 5 minutes

Cooking Time: 15 minutes

Serving: 4

Ingredients:

Three large eggs

1 cup almond flour

½ cup whole milk

Six tablespoons melted butter, divided

Two tablespoons coconut flour

One teaspoon pure vanilla extract

½ teaspoon ground cinnamon

½ teaspoon baking soda

½ teaspoon of sea salt

Directions:

Put the eggs, almond flour, milk, four tablespoons of melted butter, the coconut flour, vanilla, cinnamon, baking soda, and salt in a blender, and blend until smooth, scraping down the sides as needed.

There's something so nostalgic and comforting about pancakes. The only problem is that most are about as nutritious as a pastry—just simple starches that send you on a blood sugar roller coaster. These protein-rich pancakes have staying power and will keep you satisfied long after breakfast has ended. Top them with a handful of smashed fresh berries or a tablespoon of peanut butter.

Nutrition:

Calories: 345 - Fat: 30g - Saturated Fat: 13g - Sodium: 348mg

Total Carbohydrates: 11g - Net Carbohydrates: 6g - Fiber: 5g - Sugar: 2g

Protein: 10g

Orange Ricotta–Stuffed Crêpes

Preparation Time: 10 minutes

Cooking Time: 20 minutes

Serving: 4 (2 crêpes per person)

Ingredients:

4 ounces cream cheese, softened - Four large eggs - ½ cup almond flour

Two tablespoons coconut flour - Two teaspoons pure vanilla extract, divided

6 drops liquid stevia, divided

1 cup whole-milk ricotta cheese

One teaspoon ground cinnamon

Zest of 1 orange

Six teaspoons butter, divided

To make the crêpe batter, put the cream cheese, eggs, almond flour, coconut flour, one teaspoon of vanilla, and four drops of liquid stevia in a blender and blend until smooth, scraping down the sides as needed. Pour in just enough of the crêpe batter to evenly coat the bottom of the skillet when tilted—Cook for about 45 seconds on the first side, or until just set. Flip, and cook for 30 seconds. Carefully transfer to a plate and repeat with the remaining 4 to 5 teaspoons of butter and the remaining crêpe batter.

To serve, place about two tablespoons of ricotta mixture atop each crêpe and fold gently like an enchilada. If you have the time and are feeling fancy, after filling each crêpe with the ricotta mixture, heat a tablespoon or two of butter in the skillet, and fry each crêpe on both sides for about 1 minute, or until browned. Filled with orange-infused cinnamon ricotta, these stuffed crêpes are a meal worthy of the weekend. I'm not normally a fan of nonstick cookware, but it's essential in this recipe to produce thin crêpes that don't stick to the pan.

Nutrition:

Calories: 384g - Fat: 30g; - Saturated Fat: 15g - Sodium: 267mg - Total Carbohydrates: 12g

Net Carbohydrates: 8g - Fiber: 4g - Sugar: 1g - Protein: 18g

Cauliflower Hash Browns

Preparation Time: 15 minutes

Cooking Time: 8 to 10 minutes

Serving: 4

Ingredients:

One small head cauliflower - One teaspoon sea salt - One large egg

¼ cup shredded Parmesan cheese

Directions:

Grate the cauliflower in a food processor using the grater attachment or with the large holes of a box grater. You should have about 4 cups.

Transfer the cauliflower to a colander set over a large bowl and season with the salt. Set aside for 10 minutes.

Squeeze the cauliflower in your hands to wring out as much moisture as possible, then transfer to a large bowl.

Add the egg and Parmesan cheese, and mix until just combined.

Heat a large nonstick skillet over medium-high heat, then pour in the coconut oil, and tilt to coat the bottom.

Meanwhile, form the cauliflower into small firm patties and flatten each with your hand.

Salt draws moisture out of the cauliflower before cooking. An alternative method is to microwave the grated cauliflower for 2 to 3 minutes, let it cool, then wring it out in a clean kitchen towel or several layers of cheesecloth.

Serve these crispy, crunchy hash browns with the Green Chile Scramble for a hearty low-carb breakfast. The secret to getting the right texture with these hash browns is squeezing as much water as you can from the cauliflower.

Nutrition:

Calories: 113 - Fat: 10g - Saturated Fat: 7g - Sodium: 568mg - Total Carbohydrates: 4g

Net Carbohydrates: 2g - Fiber: 2g - Sugar: 2g - Protein: 5g

Crispy Waffles

Preparation Time: 15 minutes

Cooking Time: 20 minutes

Serves: 4

Ingredients:

½ C. super fine almond flour - ½ tsp. Swerve - ¼ tsp. Organic baking powder

¼ tsp. Baking soda - ¼ tsp. ground cinnamon - 1/8 tsp. ground cloves

1/8 tsp. Ground nutmeg - ¼ tsp. salt - Two organic eggs (whites and yolks separated)

2 tbsp. butter, melted - 1 tsp. organic vanilla extract

Directions:

In a bowl, add the flour, Swerve, baking powder, baking soda, spices, and salt and mix well.

In a second bowl, add the egg yolks, butter, and vanilla and beat until well combined.

In a third small bowl, add the egg whites and beat until soft peaks form.

Add the egg yolks mixture into the flour mixture and mix until well combined.

Gently, fold in the beaten egg whites.

Place ¼ of the mixture into preheated waffle iron and cook for about 4-5 minutes or until golden brown.

Repeat with the remaining mixture.

Serve warm.

Nutrition:

Calories per serving: 167 - Carbohydrates: 3.9g

Protein: 5.6g - Fat: 15g

Sugar: 0.8g

Sodium: 299mg

Fiber: 1.6g

CHAPTER 4:

Meat Recipes

1.   Pork Cutlets with Spanish Onion

Preparation Time: 15 minutes

Cooking Time: 15 minutes

Serving: 4

Ingredients:

One tablespoon olive oil - Two pork cutlets - One bell pepper, deveined and sliced

One Spanish onion, chopped - Two garlic cloves, minced - 1/2 teaspoon hot sauce

1/2 teaspoon mustard

1/2 teaspoon paprika

Directions:

Then, fry the pork cutlets for 3 to 4 minutes until evenly golden and crispy on both sides.

Decrease the temperature to medium and add the bell pepper, Spanish onion, garlic, hot sauce, and mustard; continue cooking until the vegetables have softened, for a further 3 minutes.

Sprinkle with paprika, salt, and black pepper. Serve immediately and enjoy!

Nutrition:

403 Calories

24.1g Fat

3.4g Total Carbs

40.1g Protein

0.7g Fiber

Rich and Easy Pork Ragout

(Ready in about 40 minutes)

Preparation Time: 15 minutes

Cooking Time: 15 minutes

Serving: 4

Ingredients:

One teaspoon lard, melted at room temperature - 3/4 pound pork butt, cut into bite-sized cubes

One red bell pepper, deveined and chopped - One poblano pepper, deveined and chopped

Two cloves garlic, pressed

1/2 cup leeks, chopped

1/2 teaspoon mustard seeds

1/4 teaspoon ground allspice

1/4 teaspoon celery seeds

1 cup roasted vegetable broth

Two vine-ripe tomatoes, pureed

Directions:

Melt the lard in a stockpot over moderate heat. Once hot, cook the pork cubes for 4 to 6 minutes, occasionally stirring to ensure even cooking.

Then, stir in the vegetables and continue cooking until they are tender and fragrant. Add in the salt, black pepper, mustard seeds, allspice, celery seeds, roasted vegetable broth, and tomatoes.

Reduce the heat to simmer. Let it simmer for 30 minutes longer or until everything is heated through.

Ladle into individual bowls and serve hot. Bon appétit!

Nutrition:

Per serving: - 389 Calories - 24.3g Fat - 5.4g Total Carbs - 33.1g Protein - 1.3g Fiber

Melt-in-Your-Mouth Pork Roast

Preparation Time: 1 hour

Cooking Time: 40 minutes

Serving: 2

Ingredients:

1 pound pork shoulder - Four tablespoons red wine

One teaspoon stone-ground mustard - One tablespoon coconut aminos

One tablespoon lemon juice - One tablespoon sesame oil

Two sprigs rosemary

One teaspoon sage

One shallot, peeled and chopped

1/2 celery stalk, chopped

1/2 head garlic, peeled and separated into cloves

Directions:

Place the pork shoulder, red wine, mustard, coconut aminos, lemon juice, sesame oil, rosemary, and sage in a ceramic dish; cover and let it marinate in your refrigerator at least 1 hour.

Discard a lightly greased baking dish. Scatter the vegetables around the pork shoulder and sprinkle with salt and black pepper.

Roast in the preheated oven at 390 degrees F for 15 minutes.

Now, reduce the temperature to 310 degrees F and continue baking an additional 40 to 45 minutes. Baste the meat with the reserved marinade once or twice.

Place on cooling racks before carving and serving. Bon appétit!

Nutrition:

497 Calories - 35.3g Fat - 2.5g Total Carbs

40.2g Protein - 0.6g Fiber

Chunky Pork Soup with Mustard Greens

Preparation Time: 25 minutes

Cooking Time: 30 minutes

Serving: 2

Ingredients:

One tablespoon olive oil - One bell pepper, deveined and chopped

Two garlic cloves, pressed - 1/2 cup scallions, chopped

1/2 pound ground pork (84% lean)- 1 cup beef bone broth

1 cup of water - 1/2 teaspoon crushed red pepper flakes

One bay laurel

One teaspoon fish sauce

2 cups mustard greens, torn into pieces

One tablespoon fresh parsley, chopped

Directions:

Coat, once hot, sauté the pepper, garlic, and scallions until tender or about 3 minutes.

After that, stir in the ground pork and cook for 5 minutes more or until well browned, stirring periodically.

Add in the beef bone broth, water, red pepper, salt, black pepper, and bay laurel. Reduce the temperature to simmer and cook, covered, for 10 minutes. Afterward, stir in the fish sauce and mustard greens.

Remove from the heat; let it stand until the greens are wilted. Ladle into individual bowls and serve garnished with fresh parsley.

Nutrition:

344 Calories - 25.2g Fat - 6.3g Total Carbs

23.1g Protein - 2.9g Fiber

Pulled Pork with Mint and Cheese

Preparation Time: 20 minutes

Cooking Time: 15 minutes

Serving: 2

Ingredients:

One teaspoon lard, melted at room temperature

3/4 pork Boston butt, sliced

Two garlic cloves, pressed

1/2 teaspoon red pepper flakes, crushed

1/2 teaspoon black peppercorns, freshly cracked

Sea salt, to taste

Two bell peppers, deveined and sliced

One tablespoon fresh mint leaves snipped

Four tablespoons cream cheese

Directions:

Melt the lard in a cast-iron skillet over a moderate flame. Once hot, brown the pork for 2 minutes per side until caramelized and crispy on the edges.

Reduce the temperature to medium-low and continue cooking another 4 minutes, turning over periodically. Shred the pork with two forks and return to the skillet.

Add the garlic, red pepper, black peppercorns, salt, and bell pepper and continue cooking for a further 2 minutes or until the peppers are just tender and fragrant.

Serve with fresh mint and a dollop of cream cheese. Enjoy!

Nutrition:

370 Calories - 21.9g Fat - 5.1g - Total Carbs - 34.9g Protein - 1g Fiber

Pork Loin Steaks in Creamy Pepper Sauce

Preparation Time: 15 minutes

Cooking Time: 10 minutes

Serving: 2

Ingredients:

One teaspoon lard, at room temperature

Two pork loin steaks

1/2 cup beef bone broth

Two bell peppers, deseeded and chopped

One shallot, chopped

One garlic clove, minced

Sea salt, to season

1/2 teaspoon cayenne pepper

1/4 teaspoon paprika

One teaspoon Italian seasoning mix

1/4 cup Greek-style yogurt

Directions:

Melt the lard in a cast-iron skillet over moderate heat. Once hot, cook the pork loin steaks until slightly browned or approximately 5 minutes per side; reserve.

Add a splash of the beef bone broth to deglaze the pan. Now, cook the bell peppers, shallot, and garlic until tender and aromatic—season with salt, cayenne pepper, paprika, and Italian seasoning mix.

After that, decrease the temperature to medium-low, add the Greek yogurt to the skillet and let it simmer for 2 minutes more or until heated through. Serve immediately.

Nutrition:

447 Calories - 19.2g Fat - 6g Total Carbs - 62.2g Protein - 1.3g Fiber

Pork Medallions with Cabbage

Preparation Time: 20 minutes

Cooking Time: 15 minutes

Serving: 2

Ingredients:

Ingredients

One ounce bacon, diced

Two pork medallions

Two garlic cloves, sliced

One red onion, chopped

One jalapeno pepper, deseeded and chopped

One tablespoon apple cider vinegar

1/2 cup chicken bone broth

1/3 pound red cabbage, shredded

One bay leaf

One sprig rosemary

One sprig thyme

Directions:

Now, cook the pork medallions in the bacon grease until they are browned on both sides.

Add the remaining ingredients and reduce the heat to medium-low. Let it cook for 13 minutes more, gently stirring periodically to ensure even cooking. Taste and adjust the seasonings.

Nutrition:

528 Calories - 31.8g Fat

6.3g Total Carbs - 51.2g Protein - 2.6g Fiber

Mom's Festive Meatloaf

Preparation Time: 1 hour

Cooking Time: 50 minutes

Serving: 2

Ingredients:

1/4 pound ground pork - 1/2 pound ground chuck

Two eggs, beaten - 1/4 cup flaxseed meal - One shallot, chopped

Two garlic cloves, minced - 1/2 teaspoon smoked paprika

1/4 teaspoon dried basil

1/4 teaspoon ground cumin

Kosher salt, to taste

1/2 cup tomato puree

One teaspoon mustard

One teaspoon liquid monk fruit

Directions:

In a mixing bowl, thoroughly combine the ground meat, eggs, flaxseed meal, shallot, garlic, and spices.

In another bowl, mix the tomato puree with the mustard and liquid monk fruit, whisk to combine well.

Press the mixture into the loaf pan—Bake in the preheated oven at 360 degrees F for 30 minutes.

Nutrition:

517 Calories - 32.3g Fat

8.4g Total Carbs - 48.5g Protein - 6.5g Fiber

Rich Winter Beef Stew

Preparation Time: 45 minutes

Cooking Time: 50 minutes

Serving: 2

Ingredients:

1-ounce bacon, diced

3/4 pound well-marbled beef chuck, boneless and cut into 1-1/2-inch pieces

One red bell pepper, chopped - One green bell pepper, chopped

Two garlic cloves, minced - 1/2 cup leeks, chopped

One parsnip, chopped - Sea salt, to taste

1/4 teaspoon mixed peppercorns, freshly cracked

2 cups of chicken bone broth

One tomato, pureed

2 cups kale, torn into pieces

One tablespoon fresh cilantro, roughly chopped

Directions:

Heat a Dutch pot over medium-high flame. Now, cook the bacon until it is well browned and crisp; reserve. Then, cook the beef pieces for 3 to 5 minutes or until just browned on all sides; reserve. After that, sauté the peppers, garlic, leeks, and parsnip in the pan drippings until they are just tender and aromatic. Add the salt, peppercorns, chicken bone broth, tomato, and reserved beef to the pot. Bring to a boil. Stir in the kale leaves and continue simmering until the leaves have wilted or 3 to 4 minutes more.

Ladle into individual bowls and serve garnished with fresh cilantro and the reserved bacon. Bon appétit!

Nutrition:

359 Calories - 17.8g Fat - 5.4g Total Carbs - 43g Protein

1g Fiber

Mini Meatloaves with Spinach

(Ready in about)

Preparation Time: 35 minutes

Cooking Time: 40 minutes

Serving: 2

Ingredients:

1/2 pound lean ground beef - Two tablespoons tomato paste

One teaspoon Dijon mustard - One egg, beaten - 1/2 teaspoon ginger garlic paste

1/2 cup shallots, finely chopped -- One tablespoon canola oil

1/2 teaspoon coconut amino - 1/4 cup almond meal

One bunch spinach, chopped

One teaspoon dried parsley flakes

1/2 teaspoon dried basil

1/2 teaspoon dried rosemary

1/2 teaspoon dried sage

1/4 teaspoon cayenne pepper

Kosher salt and ground black pepper

Two tablespoons sour cream

Directions:

Press the meat mixture into a lightly greased muffin tin. Bake the mini meatloaves in the preheated oven at 360 degrees F for 20 to 28 minutes.

Serve with sour cream and enjoy!

Nutrition:

434 Calories - 29.4g Fat - 4.4g Total Carbs - 37.1g Protein - 2.1g Fiber

CHAPTER 5:

Fish & Seafood Recipes

1.   Keto Fish

Preparation Time 40 minutes

Cooking Time: 30 minutes

Serving: 4

Ingredients:

For the Tartar Sauce

Four tablespoons dill pickle relish

1 cup mayonnaise

1/2 tablespoon curry powder

One tablespoon olive oil

1 1/2 pounds rutabaga (peeled and cleaned)

Salt and pepper, to taste

For the fish

1 1/2 pounds white fish

1 cup parmesan cheese (grated)

1 cup almond flour

Two eggs

2 cups coconut oil, for frying - One teaspoon paprika powder

1/4 teaspoon pepper - 1/2 teaspoon onion powder - One lemon

One teaspoon salt

Directions:

Take a small bowl and mix mayonnaise, curry powder, and pickle relish thoroughly. Refrigerate the tartar sauce until you finish the remaining dish.

Preheat the oven to 400 degrees Fahrenheit.

Slice the peeled rutabaga into thin rods and brush them with oil.

Line a baking tray with parchment paper and spread the oil-coated rutabaga rods.

Sprinkle the pepper and salt over the spread rutabaga.

Bake for 30 minutes until the rods become golden brown.

As the rutabaga gets cooked, Preparation, the fish.

Crack the eggs into a small bowl and beat it well with a fork.

Mix the Parmesan cheese, almond flour, paprika powder, pepper, onion powder, and salt on a plate. Set aside.

Dip the flour-coated fix into the beaten eggs and coat it again with the flour mix.

Pour the oil in a shallow skillet and heat over high heat.

If the rutabaga chips are ready by now, turn off the oven and let it sit for a while.

Fry the flour-egg coated fish in the hot oil until the fish is completely cooked and turns golden brown.

Repeat steps 11 and 14 with the remaining fish.

Transfer the fried fish, baked rutabaga fries, and tartar into a serving bowl.

Serve hot and enjoy!

Nutrition:

Calories 463 Kcal

Fat: 26.2 g

Protein: 49.2 g

Net carb: 4 g

Zingy Lemon Fish

Preparation Time 50 minutes

Cooking Time: 40 minutes

Serving: 4

Ingredients:

14 ounces fresh Gurnard fish fillets

Two tablespoons lemon juice

Six tablespoons butter

½ cup fine almond flour

Two teaspoons dried chives

One teaspoon garlic powder

Two teaspoons dried dill

Two teaspoons onion powder

Salt and pepper to taste

Directions:

Add almond flour, dried herbs, salt, and spices on a large plate and stir until well combined. Spread it all over the plate evenly.

Place a large pan over medium-high heat. Add half the butter and half the lemon juice. When butter just melts, place fillets on the pan and cook for 3 minutes. Move the fillets around the pan so that it absorbs the butter and lemon juice.

Add remaining half butter and lemon juice. When butter melts, flip sides and cook the other side for 3 minutes.

Serve fillets with any butter remaining in the pan.

Nutrition:

Calories 406 Kcal - Fat: 30.33 g

Protein: 29 g - Net carb: 3.55 g

Creamy Keto Fish Casserole

Preparation Time 1 hour

Cooking Time: 50 minutes

Serving: 4

Ingredients:

25 ounces of white fish (slice into bite-sized pieces)

15 ounces broccoli (small florets, include the step too) - 3 ounces butter + extra

Six scallions (finely chopped) - 1 1/4 cups heavy whipping cream - Two tablespoons small capers

One tablespoon dried parsley - One tablespoon Dijon mustard

1/4 teaspoon black pepper (ground) - One teaspoon salt - Two tablespoons olive oil

5 ounces leafy greens (finely chopped), for garnishing

Directions:

Preheat the oven to 400 degrees Fahrenheit. Heat the oil in a saucepan over medium-high heat.

Fry the broccoli florets in the hot oil for 5 minutes until tender and golden.

Transfer the fried florets to a small bowl and season it with salt and pepper. Toss the contents to ensure all the florets get an equal amount of seasoning.

Add the chopped scallions and capers to the same saucepan and fry for 2 minutes. Return the florets to the pan and mix well.

Grease a baking tray with a little amount of butter and spread the fried veggies (broccoli, scallions, and capers) in the baking tray.

Add the sliced fish to the tray and nestle it among the veggies.

Mix the heavy cream, mustard, and parsley in a small bowl and pour this mixture over the fish-veggie mixture. Top this with the remaining butter and spread gently over the contents using a spatula. Transfer to a plate and garnish with chopped greens. Serve warm and enjoy!

Nutrition:

Calories 822 - Kcal Fat: 69 g - Protein: 41 g - Net carb: 8 g

Keto Fish Casserole With Mushrooms And French Mustard

Preparation Time 1 hour

Cooking Time: 50 minutes

Serving: 6

Ingredients:

25 ounces of white fish - 15 ounces mushrooms (cut into wedges)

20 ounces cauliflower (cut into florets) - 2 cups heavy whipping cream - 3 ounces butter

Two tablespoons Dijon mustard - 3 ounces olive oil - 8 ounces cheese (shredded)

Two tablespoons fresh parsley

Salt & pepper, to taste

Directions:

Preheat the oven to 350 degrees Fahrenheit

Fry the mushroom for 5 minutes until tender and soft.

Add the parsley, salt, and pepper to the mushrooms as you continue to mix well.

Reduce the heat and add the mustard and heavy whipping cream to the mushroom.

Allow it simmer for 10 minutes until the sauce thickens and reduces a bit.

Season the fish slices with pepper and salt. Set aside.

9. Sprinkle 3/4th of the cheese over the fish slices and spread the creamy mushroom over the top. Now again, top it with the remaining cheese.

Boil the cauliflower florets in lightly salted water for 5 minutes and strain the water.

Place the strained florets in a bowl and add the olive oil. Mash thoroughly with a fork until you get a coarse texture—season with salt and pepper. Mix well.

Nutrition:

Calories 828 - Fat: 71 g

Protein: 39 g - Net carb: 8 g

Keto Thai Fish With Curry And Coconut

Preparation Time 50 minutes

Cooking Time: 40 minutes

Serving: 4

Ingredients:

25 ounces salmon (slice into bite-sized pieces)

15 ounces cauliflower (bite-sized florets)

14 ounces coconut cream

1-ounce olive oil

Four tablespoons butter

Salt and pepper, to taste

Directions:

Preheat the oven to 400 degrees Fahrenheit

Sprinkle salt and pepper over the salmon generously. Toss it once, if possible.

Place the butter generously over all the salmon pieces and set aside.

Pour this cream mixture over the fish in the baking tray.

Meanwhile, boil the cauliflower florets in salted water for 5 minutes, strain and mash the florets coarsely. Set aside.

Transfer the creamy fish to a plate and serve with mashed cauliflower. Enjoy!

Nutrition:

Calories 880 Kcal

Fat: 75 g

Protein: 42 g

Net carb: 6 g)

Keto Salmon Tandoori With Cucumber Sauce
Servings: 4

Ingredients

25 ounces salmon (bite-sized pieces) - Two tablespoons coconut oil

One tablespoon tandoori seasoning

For the cucumber sauce

1/2 shredded cucumber (squeeze out the water completely) - Juice of 1/2 lime

Two minced garlic cloves - 1 1/4 cups sour cream or mayonnaise

1/2 teaspoon salt (optional)

For the crispy salad

3 1/2 ounces lettuce (torn) - Three scallions (finely chopped)

Two avocados (cubed) - One yellow bell pepper (diced) - Juice of 1 lime

Directions:

Preheat the oven to 350 degrees Fahrenheit

Mix the tandoori seasoning with oil in a small bowl and coat the salmon pieces with this mixture.

Bake for 20 minutes until soft and the salmon flakes with a fork

Take another bowl and place the shredded cucumber in it. Add the mayonnaise, minced garlic, and salt (if the mayonnaise doesn't have salt) to the shredded cucumber.

Mix the lettuce, scallions, avocados, and bell pepper in another bowl. Drizzle the contents with the lime juice.

Transfer the veggie salad to a plate and place the baked salmon over it. Top the veggies and salmon with cucumber sauce.

Serve immediately and enjoy!

Nutrition:

Calories 847 Kcal - Fat: 73 g - Protein: 35 g - Net carb: 6 g

Creamy Mackerel

This is creamy and rich!

Preparation time: 10 minutes

Cooking time: 20 minutes

Servings: 4

Ingredients:

Two shallots, minced

Two spring onions, chopped

Two tablespoons olive oil

Four mackerel fillets, skinless and cut into medium cubes

1 cup heavy cream

One teaspoon cumin, ground

½ teaspoon oregano, dried

A pinch of salt and black pepper

Two tablespoons chives, chopped

Directions:

Heat a pan with the oil over medium heat, add the spring onions and the shallots, stir and sauté for 5 minutes.

Add the fish and cook it for 4 minutes.

Add the rest of the ingredients, bring to a simmer, cook everything for 10 minutes more, divide between plates, and serve.

Nutrition:

Calories 403 - Fat 33.9 - Fiber 0.4

Carbs 2.7 - Protein 22

Lime Mackerel

It's an easy keto dish for you to enjoy tonight for dinner!

Preparation Time: 10 Minutes

Cooking Time: 30 Minutes

Servings: 4

Ingredients:

Four mackerel fillets, boneless

Two tablespoons lime juice

Two tablespoons olive oil

A pinch of salt and black pepper

½ teaspoon sweet paprika

Directions:

Arrange the mackerel on a baking sheet lined with parchment paper, add the oil and the other ingredients, rub gently, introduce in the oven at 360 degrees F and bake for 30 minutes.

Divide the fish between plates and serve.

Nutrition:

Calories 297

Fat 22.7

Fiber 0.2

Carbs 2

Protein 21.1

Turmeric Tilapia

This great dish is perfect for a special evening!

Preparation time: 10 minutes

Cooking time: 12 minutes

Servings: 4

Ingredients:

Four tilapia fillets, boneless

Two tablespoons olive oil

One teaspoon turmeric powder

A pinch of salt and black pepper

Two spring onions, chopped

¼ teaspoon basil, dried

¼ teaspoon garlic powder

One tablespoon parsley, chopped

Directions:

Heat a pan with the oil over medium heat, add the spring onions and cook them for 2 minutes.

Add the fish, turmeric, and the other ingredients, cook for 5 minutes on each side, divide between plates and serve.

Nutrition:

Calories 205

Fat 8.6

Fiber 0.4

Carbs 1.1

Protein 31.8

Walnut Salmon Mix

You just have to try this wonderful combination!

Preparation Time: 10 Minutes

Cooking Time: 14 Minutes

Servings: 4

Ingredients:

Four salmon fillets, boneless

Two tablespoons avocado oil

A pinch of salt and black pepper

One tablespoon lime juice

Two shallots, chopped

Two tablespoons walnuts, chopped

Two tablespoons parsley, chopped

Directions:

Heat a pan with the oil over medium-high heat, add the shallots, stir and sauté for 2 minutes.

Add the fish and the other ingredients, cook for 6 minutes on each side, divide between plates and serve.

Nutrition:

Calories 276

Fat 14.2

Fiber 0.7

Carbs 2.7

Protein 35.8

Chives Trout

The fish is so rich and flavored!

Preparation Time: 10 Minutes

Cooking Time: 12 Minutes

Servings: 4

Ingredients:

Four trout fillets, boneless

Two shallots, chopped

A pinch of salt and black pepper

Three tablespoons chives, chopped

Two tablespoons avocado oil

Two teaspoons lime juice

Directions:

Heat a pan with the oil over medium heat, add the shallots and sauté them for 2 minutes.

Add the fish and the rest of the ingredients, cook for 5 minutes on each side, divide between plate sand serve.

Nutrition:

Calories 320

Fat 12

Fiber 1

Carbs 2

Protein 24

Salmon and Tomatoes

Feel free to serve this great dish today1

Preparation Time: 10 Minutes

Cooking Time: 25 Minutes

Servings: 4

Ingredients:

Two tablespoons avocado oil

Four salmon fillets, boneless

1 cup cherry tomatoes, halved

Two spring onions, chopped

½ cup chicken stock

A pinch of salt and black pepper

½ teaspoon rosemary, dried

Directions:

In a roasting pan, combine the fish with the oil and the other ingredients, introduce in the oven at 400 degrees F and bake for 25 minutes.

Divide between plates and serve.

Nutrition:

calories 200

fat 12

fiber 0

carbs 3

protein 21

CHAPTER 6:

Vegetables And Salad Recipes

1.   Roasted Brussels Sprouts Salad with Parmesan

The difference between this dish and most roasted Brussels sprouts is that here we are just using the leaves of the sprouts, which makes the dish super light. Hazelnuts are not an ingredient I use often, but they play a starring role in this salad.

Preparation Time 10 minutes

Cooking Time: 15 minutes

Serving: 2

Ingredients:

1 pound Brussels sprouts - One tablespoon olive oil - Pink Himalayan salt

Freshly ground black pepper - ¼ cup shaved or grated Parmesan cheese

¼ cup whole, skinless hazelnuts

Directions:

Preheat the oven to 350°F. Line a baking sheet with a silicone baking mat or parchment paper. Trim the bottom and core from each Brussels sprout with a small knife. This will release the leaves. (You can reserve the cores to roast later if you wish.). Put the leaves in a medium bowl; you can use your hands to release all the leaves fully. Toss the leaves with the olive oil and season with pink Himalayan salt and pepper. Spread the leaves in a single layer on the baking sheet—roast for 10 to 15 minutes, or until lightly browned and crisp. Divide the roasted Brussels sprouts leaves between two bowls, top each with the shaved Parmesan cheese and hazelnuts, and serve.

If you don't have hazelnuts, use chopped almonds.

Nutrition:

Calories: 287 - Total Fat: 19g - Carbs: 23g - Net Carbs: 13g - Fiber: 10g - Protein: 14g

Wedge Salad

To me, a crisp iceberg lettuce wedge topped with chunky blue cheese dressing is delicious on its own. But when you add juicy grape tomatoes and crunchy bacon? It's just perfect.

Preparation Time 10 minutes

Cooking Time: 10 minutes

Serving: 2

Ingredients:

Four bacon slices

½ head iceberg lettuce halved

Two tablespoons blue cheese salad dressing (I use Trader Joe's Chunky Blue Cheese Dressing)

¼ cup blue cheese crumbles

½ cup halved grape tomatoes

Directions:

In a large skillet over medium-high heat, cook the bacon on both sides until crispy, about 8 minutes. Transfer the bacon to a paper towel-lined plate to drain and cool for 5 minutes. Transfer to a cutting board and chop the bacon.

Place the lettuce wedges on two plates. Top each with half of the blue cheese dressing, the blue cheese crumbles, the halved grape tomatoes, and the chopped bacon, and serve.

If you have a grill, you can drizzle each of your iceberg lettuce wedges with one tablespoon of olive oil, season with pink Himalayan salt and pepper, and grill each side for about 1 minute to add some smoky flavor. Then dress the lettuce wedges as instructed.

Nutrition:

Calories: 278 - Total Fat: 20g

Carbs: 9g - Net Carbs: 7g

Fiber: 3g - Protein: 15g

Mexican Egg Salad

I have always been a big fan of egg salad. It also makes a great base for experimentation with different flavors and textures. This version of avocado egg salad brings fresh cilantro and diced jalapeños to the party for a little kick. Then for some crunch, let's put the egg salad on cheese chips! For additional zest, add ½ teaspoon of Tajín seasoning salt and the juice of ½ a lime to the egg salad.

Preparation Time 15 minutes

Cooking Time: 10 minutes

Serving: 2

Ingredients:

Four large eggs - ½ cup shredded cheese (I use Mexican blend), divided

One jalapeño - One avocado halved - Pink Himalayan salt

Freshly ground black pepper - Two tablespoons chopped fresh cilantro

Directions:

Preheat the oven to 350°F. Line a baking sheet with parchment paper or a silicone baking mat. To Make The Hardboiled Eggs. In a medium saucepan, cover the eggs with water. Place over high heat, and bring the water to a boil. Once it is boiling, turn off the heat, cover, and leave on the burner for 10 to 12 minutes. Use a slotted spoon to remove the eggs from the pan and run them under cold water for 1 minute or submerge in an ice bath. Gently tap the shells and peel. (I like to run cold water over my hands as I peel the shells off.). To Make The Cheese Chips

While the eggs are cooking, put 2 (¼-cup) mounds of shredded cheese on the prepared pan and bake for about 7 minutes, or until the edges are brown and the middle has fully melted.

Remove the cheese chips from the oven and allow to cool for 5 minutes; they will be floppy when they first come out but will crisp as they cool. In a medium bowl, chop the hardboiled eggs.

Stem, rib, seed, and dice the jalapeño and add it to the eggs. Mash the avocado with a fork—season with pink Himalayan salt and pepper. Add the avocado and cilantro to the eggs and stir to combine.

Place the cheese chips on two plates, top with the egg salad, and serve.

Nutrition:

Calories: 359 - Total Fat: 29g - Carbs: 8g - Net Carbs: 3g - Fiber: 5g - Protein: 21g

Blue Cheese and Bacon Kale Salad

I love a massaged kale salad. Massaging the kale leaves with olive oil breaks down the fibers and makes the greens more tender and easier to digest. Top the kale with bacon, blue cheese crumbles, and pecans, and you have a nutritious salad packed with unique flavors and textures.

Preparation Time 10 minutes

Cooking Time: 10 minutes

Serving: 2

Ingredients:

Four bacon slices

2 cups stemmed and chopped fresh kale

One tablespoon vinaigrette salad dressing (I use Primal Kitchen Greek Vinaigrette)

Pinch pink Himalayan salt

Pinch freshly ground black pepper

¼ cup pecans

¼ cup blue cheese crumbles

In a medium skillet over medium-high heat, cook the bacon on both sides until crispy, about 8 minutes. Transfer the bacon to a paper towel-lined plate.

Meanwhile, in a large bowl, massage the kale with the vinaigrette for 2 minutes. Add the pink Himalayan salt and pepper. Let the kale sit while the bacon cooks, and it will get even softer.

Chop the bacon and pecans, and add them to the bowl. Sprinkle in the blue cheese.

Toss well to combine, portion onto two plates, and serve.

Chopped almonds can replace the chopped pecans.

Nutrition:

Calories: 353 - Total Fat: 29g

Carbs: 10g - Net Carbs: 7g

Fiber: 3g - Protein: 16g

Chopped Greek Salad

A Greek salad is one of my restaurant favorites. It is so fresh and easy to make. This one has just a few ingredients, but feel free to get creative with yours.

Preparation Time 10 minutes

Cooking Time: 10 minutes

Serving: 2

Ingredients:

2 cups chopped romaine - ½ cup halved grape tomatoes - ¼ cup sliced black olives (like Kalamata)

¼ cup feta cheese crumbles

Two tablespoons vinaigrette salad dressing (I use Primal Kitchen Greek Vinaigrette)

Pink Himalayan salt

Freshly ground black pepper

One tablespoon olive oil

Directions:

In a large bowl, combine the romaine, tomatoes, olives, feta cheese, and vinaigrette.

Season with pink Himalayan salt and pepper, drizzle with the olive oil and toss to combine.

Divide the salad between two bowls and serve.

VARIATIONS

With Greek salad, there are so many great flavors you can add:

Red onion or finely chopped cucumbers for additional crunch and freshness, and chopped pepperoncini for a zesty kick.

Finely chopped Genoa salami and pepperoni are good choices.

You could replace the feta cheese with goat cheese.

Nutrition:

Calories: 202 - Total Fat: 19g - Carbs: 4g - Net Carbs: 3g - Fiber: 2g - Protein: 4g

Mediterranean Cucumber Salad

I love making this salad because it is so simple, so delicious, and so packed with fresh flavors. The black olives and feta cheese add some healthy fats, while the cucumbers and tomatoes add that pop of freshness—a great side salad for any Mediterranean-inspired meat dish.

Preparation Time 10 minutes

Cooking Time: 15 minutes

Serving: 2

Ingredients:

One large cucumber, peeled and finely chopped

½ cup halved grape tomatoes

¼ cup halved black olives (I used Kalamata)

¼ cup crumbled feta cheese

Pink Himalayan salt

Directions:

Freshly ground black pepper

Two tablespoons vinaigrette salad dressing (I use Primal Kitchen Greek Vinaigrette)

In a large bowl, combine the cucumber, tomatoes, olives, and feta cheese—season with pink Himalayan salt and pepper. Add the dressing and toss to combine.

Divide the salad between two bowls and serve.

This salad can be eaten immediately, of course, but I think it is even better if you cover it with wrap and put it in the fridge to let the dressing marinate the salad ingredients for a few hours.

Nutrition:

Per Serving - Calories: 152

Total Fat: 13g

Carbs: 6g - Net Carbs: 4g - Fiber: 2g - Protein: 4g

Avocado Egg Salad Lettuce Cups

I just recently started making egg salad with avocado instead of mayo. It adds a delicious flavor element. And for some enjoyable crunch, add sliced radishes.

Preparation Time 15 minutes

Cooking Time: 15 minutes

Serving: 2

Ingredients:

Four large eggs

One avocado halved

Pink Himalayan salt

Freshly ground black pepper

½ teaspoon freshly squeezed lemon juice

Four butter lettuce cups washed and patted dry with paper towels or a clean dish towel

Two radishes, thinly sliced

Directions:

TO MAKE THE HARDBOILED EGGS

1. In a medium saucepan, cover the eggs with water. Place over high heat, and bring the water to a boil. Once it is boiling, turn off the heat, cover, and leave on the burner for 10 to 12 minutes.

2. Remove the eggs with a slotted spoon and run them under cold water for 1 minute or submerge them in an ice bath.

3. Then gently tap the shells and peel. Run cold water over your hands as you remove the shells.

TO MAKE THE EGG SALAD

1. In a medium bowl, chop the hardboiled eggs.

2. Add the avocado to the bowl, and mash the flesh with a fork. Season with pink Himalayan salt and pepper, add the lemon juice and stir to combine.

3. Place the four lettuce cups on two plates. Top the lettuce cups with the egg salad and the slices of radish and serve.

VARIATIONS

For this recipe, you can incorporate additional ingredients that you may have in your refrigerator or pantry:

Add a guacamole vibe to your egg salad with chopped jalapeño and red onion.

Chopped bacon adds appealing texture to your egg salad, or add slices of crisp bacon to your lettuce cups.

You could also use romaine hearts or baby cos lettuce.

Nutrition:

Calories: 258

Total Fat: 20g

Carbs: 8g

Net Carbs: 3g

Fiber: 5g

Protein: 15g

CHAPTER 7:

Soup Recipes

1.   Creamy Broccoli and Leek Soup

This one appetizer is perfect for any dinner or lunch, mostly the last one, but you can't go wrong using it any time of the day.

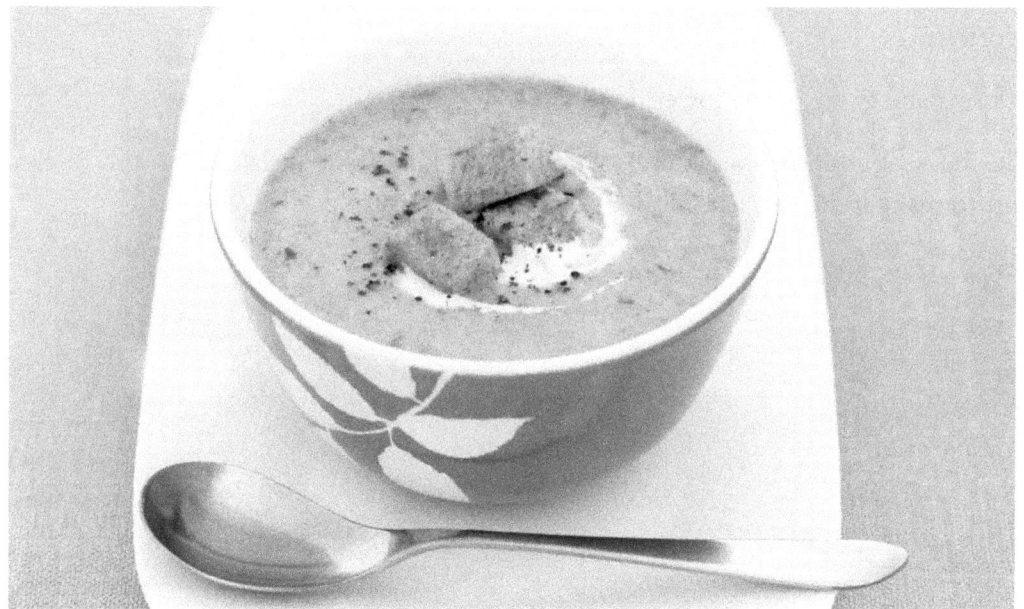

Preparation time: 5 minutes

Cooking time: 25 minutes

Servings: 4

Ingredients:

Ten ozs. broccoli

One leek

Eight ozs. cream cheese

Three ozs. butter

3 cups of water

One garlic clove

½ cup fresh basil

salt and pepper

Directions:

Rinse the leek and chop both parts finely. Slice the broccoli thinly.

Place the veggies in a pot and cover with water and then season them. Boil the water until the broccoli softens.

Add the florets and garlic, while lowering the heat.

Add in the cheese, butter, pepper, and basil. Blend until desired consistency: if too thick use water; if you want to make it thicker, use a little bit of heavy cream.

Nutrition:

Calories: 451 kcal

Fats: 37 g

Protein: 10 g

Carbs: 4 g

Chicken Soup

When you are talking about soups, what's the first thing that enters your mind? Chicken soup, of course. So there is no way we could leave this out this one!

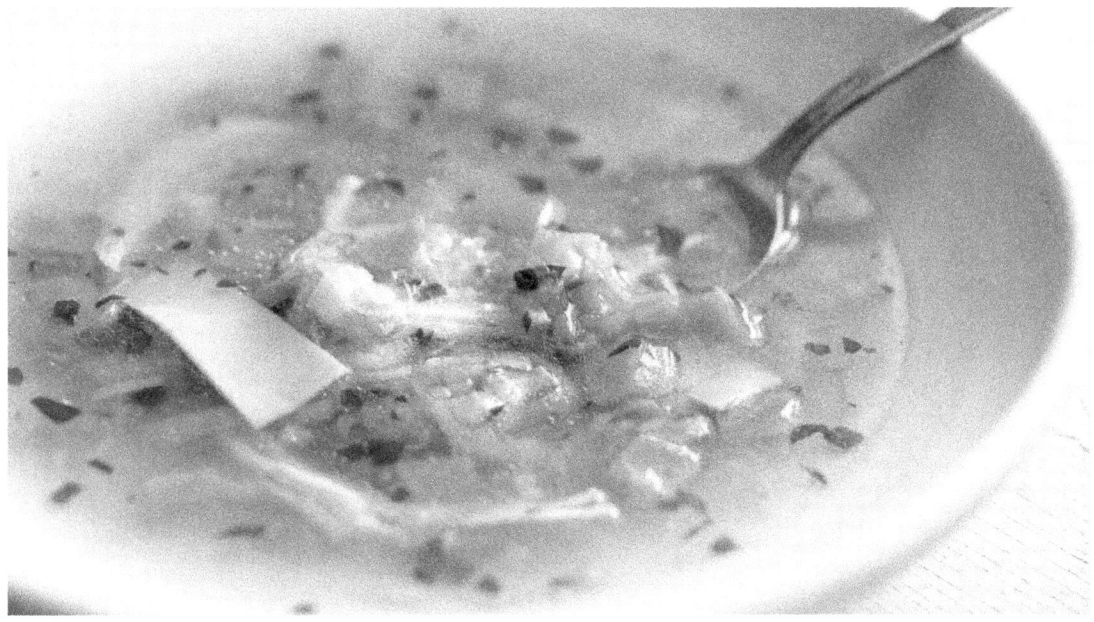

Preparation time: 25 minutes

Cooking time: 80 mins

Servings: 4

Ingredients:

6 cups of water

One chicken

One medium carrot

One yellow onion

One bay leaf

One leek

Two garlic cloves

1 tbsp. dried thyme

½ cup white wine, dry (no, not for drinking)

1 tsp. peppercorns

salt and pepper

Directions:

Peel and cut your veggies. Brown them in oil in a big pot.

Split your chicken in half, down in the middle. Pour water and spices in the pot. Let it simmer for one hour.

Take out the chicken, save the meat, and toss away the bones.

Put the meat back in the pot, and let it simmer on medium heat for 20-25 mins again, while seasoning to your liking.

Nutrition:

Calories: 145 kcal

Fats: 12 g

Carbs: 1 g

Protein: 8 g

Greek Egg and Lemon Soup with Chicken

If you want something refreshing and Mediterranean, then this soup will suit you perfectly!

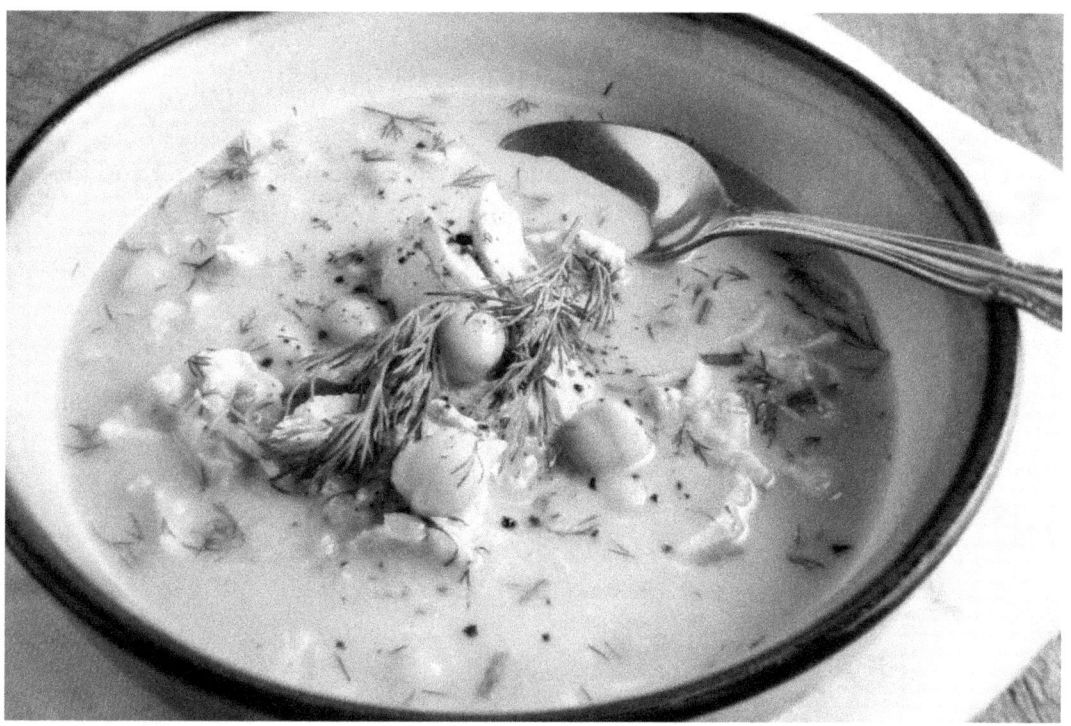

Preparation time: 5 minutes

Cooking time: 30 minutes

Servings: 4

Ingredients:

4 cups of water

¾ lbs. cauli

1 lb. boneless chicken thighs

1/3 lb. butter

Four eggs

One lemon

2 tbsps. fresh parsley

One bay leaf

Two chicken bouillon cubes

salt and pepper

Directions:

Slice your chicken thinly and then place it in a saucepan while adding cold water and the cubes and bay leaf. Let the meat simmer for 10 mins before removing it and the bay leaf.

Grate your cauli and place it in a saucepan. Add butter and boil for a few minutes.

Beat your eggs and lemon juice in a bowl, while seasoning it.

Reduce the heat a bit and add the eggs, stirring continuously. Let simmer but don't boil.

Return the chicken.

Nutrition:

Calories: 582 kcal

Carbs: 4 g

Fats: 49 g

Protein: 31 g

Wild Mushroom Soup

Mushrooms are so good for every dish, but our favorite is a bowl of creamy soup. This soup is smooth and satisfying, just as everything in life should be!

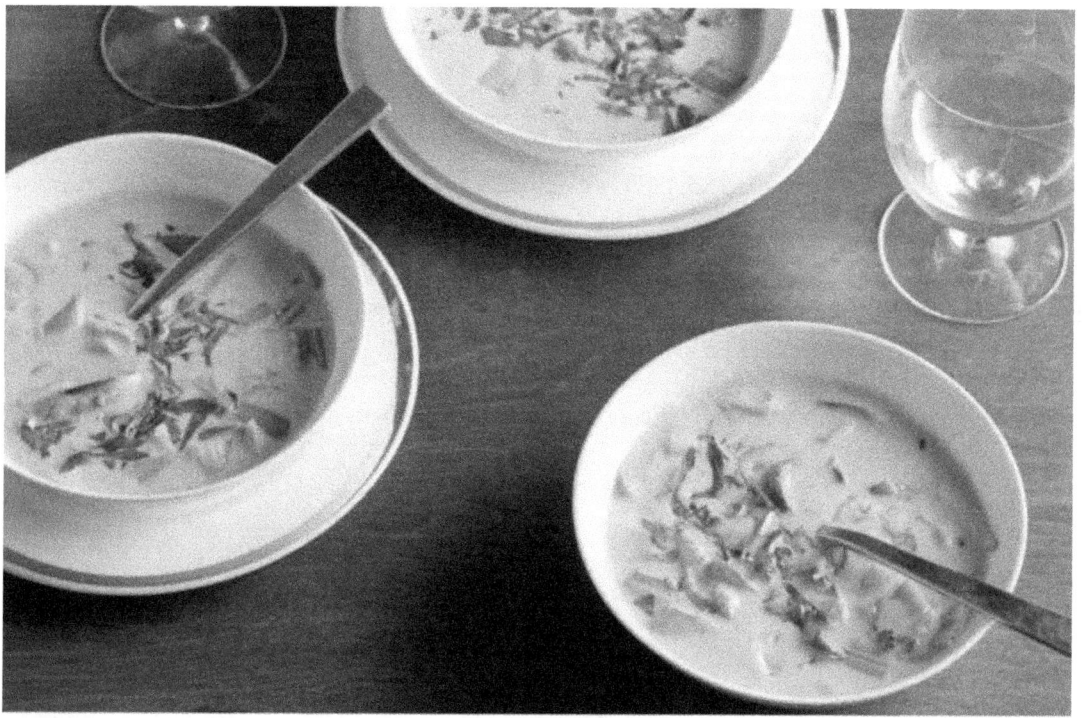

Preparation Time: 10 mins

Cooking Time: 30 mins

Servings: 4

Ingredients:

Six ozs. the mix of portabella mushrooms, oyster mushrooms, and shiitake mushrooms

3 cups of water

One garlic clove

One shallot

Four ozs. butter

One chicken bouillon cube

½ lb. celery root

1 tbsp. white wine vinegar

1 cup heavy whipping cream

fresh parsley

Directions:

Clean, trim, and chop your mushrooms and celery. Do the same to your shallot and garlic.

Sauté your chopped veggies in butter over medium heat in a saucepan.

Add thyme, vinegar, chicken bouillon cube, and water as you bring to boil. Then let it simmer for 10-15 mins.

Add cream to them with an immersion blender until your desired consistency. Serve with parsley on top.

Nutrition:

Calories: 481 kcal

Fats: 47 g

Protein: 7 g

Carbs: 9 g

Roasted Butternut Squash Soup

This one is a little bit longer soup, based on its cooking time, but it's worth it, trust us. When you roast it and inhale the caramelized smell, you will know that you made the right choice.

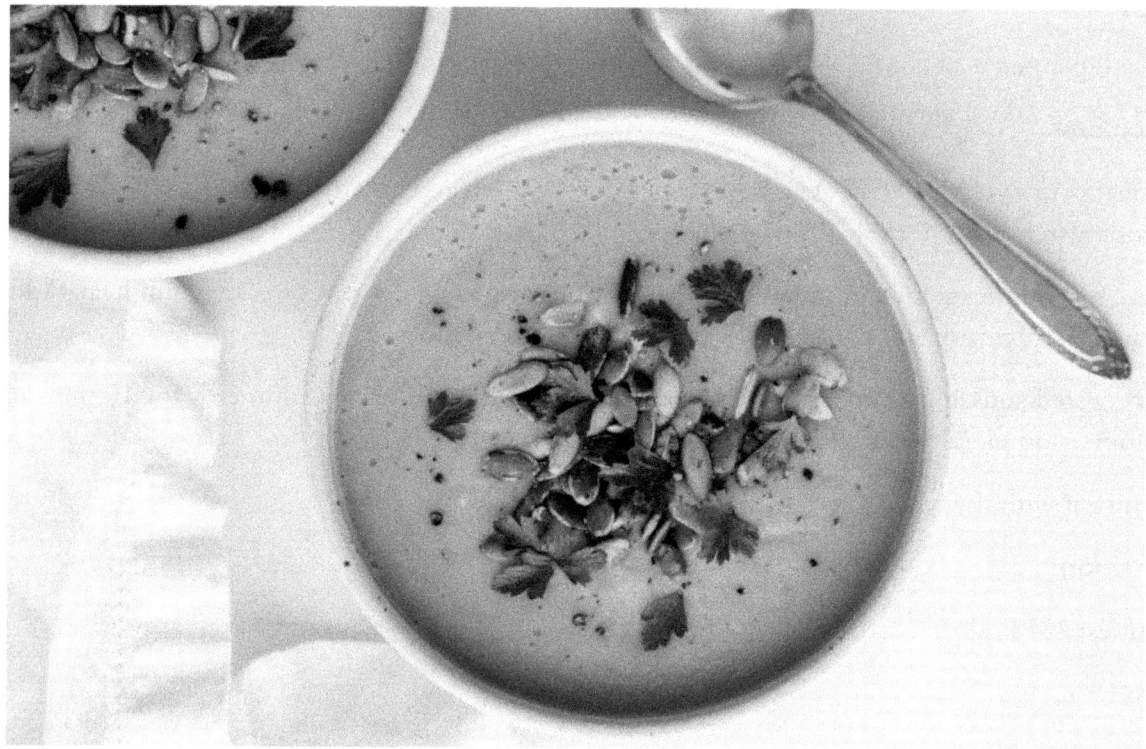

Preparation Time: 15 minutes

Cooking Time: 30 minutes

Servings: 4

Ingredients:

One large butternut squash, cubed and peeled

One stalk celery, sliced

Two potatoes, peeled, chopped

One onion, chopped

One large carrot, chopped

3 tbsps. olive oil

1 tbsp. fresh thyme

25 ozs. chicken broth

1 tbsp. butter

salt and pepper

Directions:

Preheat your oven to 400°F. On a baking sheet, toss squash and potatoes with 2 tbsp. Oil and season to your taster. Roast for 20-25 mins.

In the meantime, melt your butter and the rest of the oil in a large pot over medium heat. Add the onion, celery, carrot, and cook for 5-8 mins. Season them, too.

Add roasted squash and potatoes. Then pour over the chicken broth. Simmer it for 10 mins using an immersion blender until the soup is creamy.

Garnish it with thyme.

Nutrition:

Calories: 254 kcal

Fats: 15 g

Carbs: 19 g

Protein: 6 g

Zucchini Cream Soup

Zucchini is often the forgotten veggie. So, with this creamy and easy soup, we are here to show you the worth of this gorgeous green stuff.

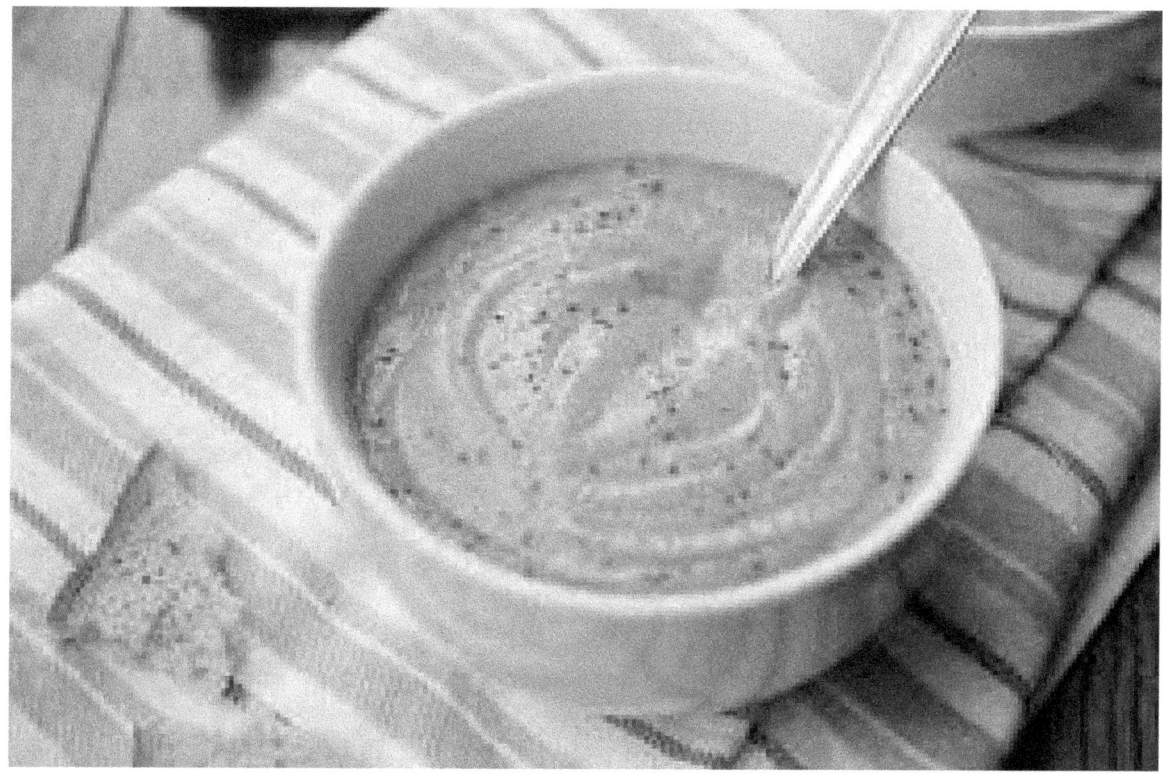

Preparation Time: 5 minutes

Cooking Time: 20 minutes

Servings: 4

Ingredients:

Three zucchinis

32 ozs. chicken broth

Two cloves garlic

2 tbsps. sour cream

½ small onion

parmesan cheese (for topping if desired)

Directions:

Combine your broth, garlic, zucchini, and onion in a large pot over medium heat until boiling.

Lower the heat, cover, and let simmer for 15-20 mins

Remove from heat and purée with an immersion blender while adding the sour cream and pureeing until smooth.

Season to taste and top with your cheese.

Nutrition:

Calories: 117 kcal

Fats: 9 g

Carbs: 3 g

Protein: 4 g

Cauli Soup

As you already know, we are a fan of cauliflower; so of course, there will be soup in front of it. But don't worry, this is just as delicious as every other cauli meal that we've already shown, so t you won't be disappointed.

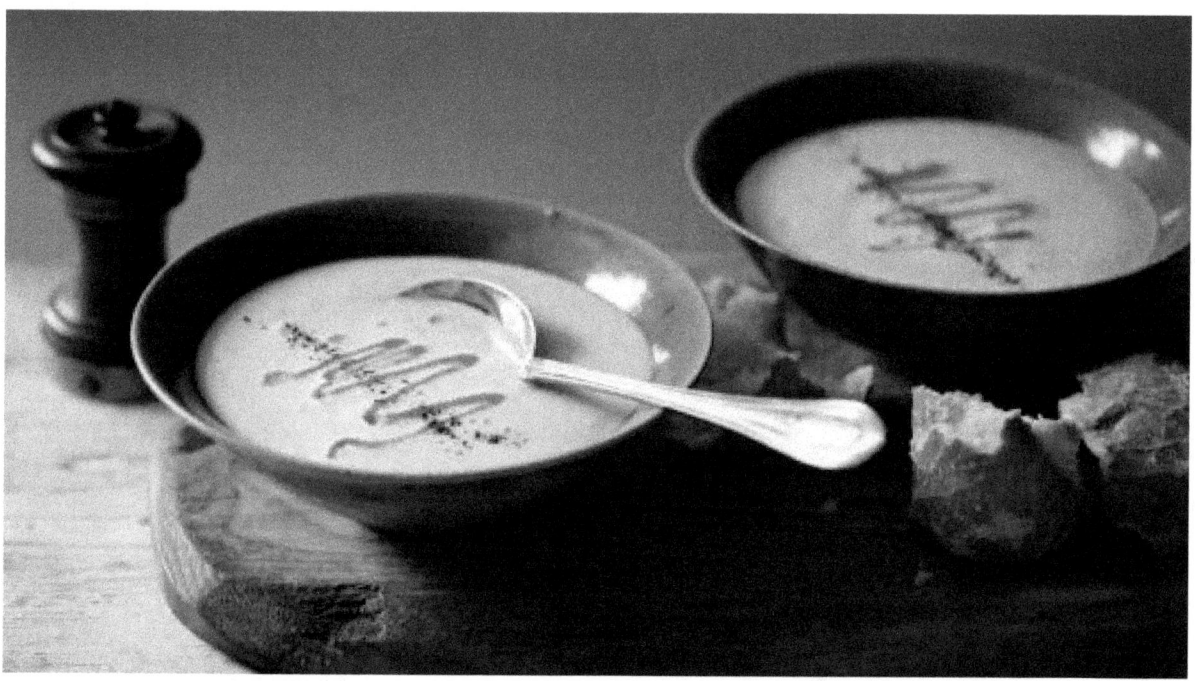

Preparation Time: 5 minutes

Cooking Time: 25 minutes

Servings: 6

Ingredients:

32 ozs. vegetable broth

One head cauli, diced

Two garlic cloves, minced

One onion, diced

½ tbsp. olive oil

salt and pepper

grated parmesan, sliced green onion for topping

Directions:

In a pot, heat oil over medium heat, while adding the onion and garlic. Then cook them for 4-5 mins.

Add in the cauli and vegetable broth. Boil it and then cover for 15-20 mins while covered.

Pour all contents of the pot into a blender and season it.

Blend until smooth. Top it with your cheese and green onion.

Nutrition:

Calories: 37 kcal

Fats: 1 g

Carbs: 3 g

Protein: 3 g

Thai Coconut Soup

Thailand is a dream place for almost everyone, so we are bringing you a really small piece of it to your diet since you deserve a holiday!

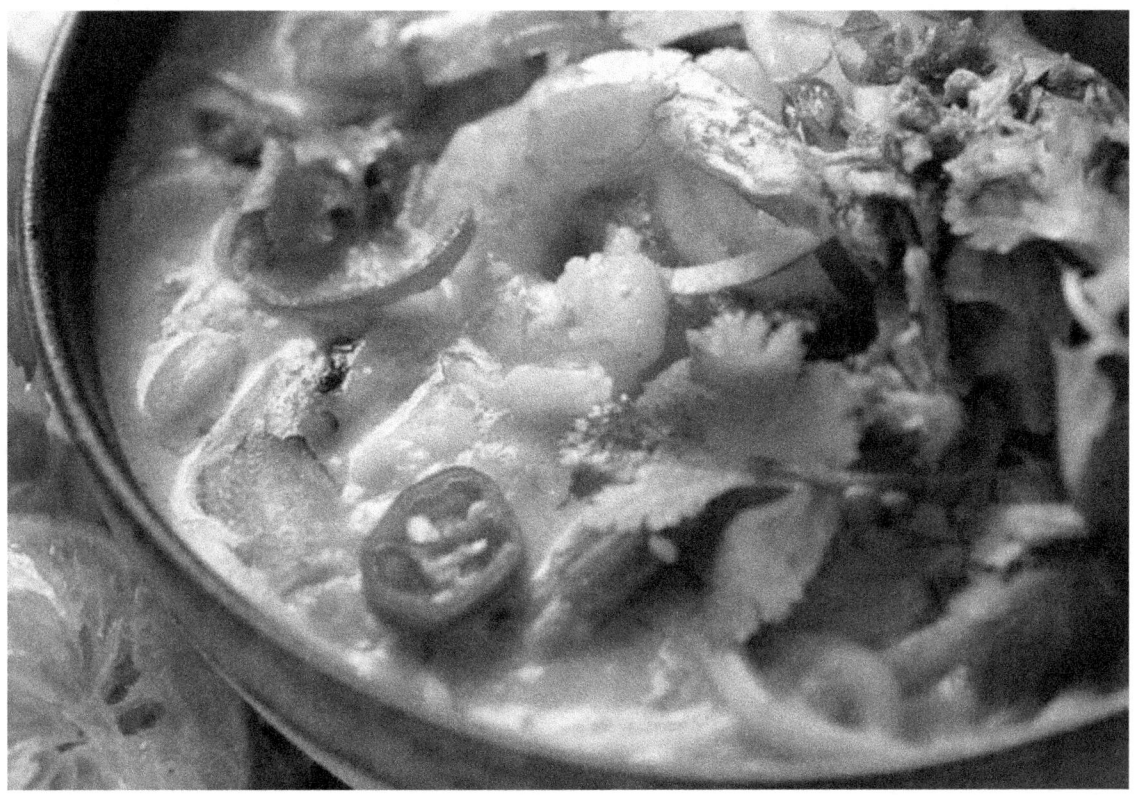

Preparation Time: 10 Minutes

Cooking Time: 35 Minutes

Servings: 4

Ingredients:

Three chicken breasts

Nine ozs. coconut milk

Nine ozs. chicken broth

2/3 tbsps. chili sauce

18 ozs. water

2/3 tbsps. coconut aminos

2/3 ozs. lime juice

2/3 tsp. ground ginger

¼ cup red boat fish sauce

salt and pepper

Directions:

Slice up the chicken breasts thinly. Make them bite-sized.

In a large stockpot, mix your coconut milk, water, fish sauce, chili sauce, lime juice, ginger, coconut aminos, and broth. Bring to a boil.

Stir in chicken pieces. Then reduce the heat and cover pot, while simmering it for 30 mins.

Remove the basil leaves and season it.

Nutrition:

Calories: 227 kcal

Fats: 17 g

Carbs: 3 g

Protein: 19 g

Chicken Ramen Soup

Ramen is one of those soups which can be used as a main dish. We are giving you a lighter version, but it's still really filling.

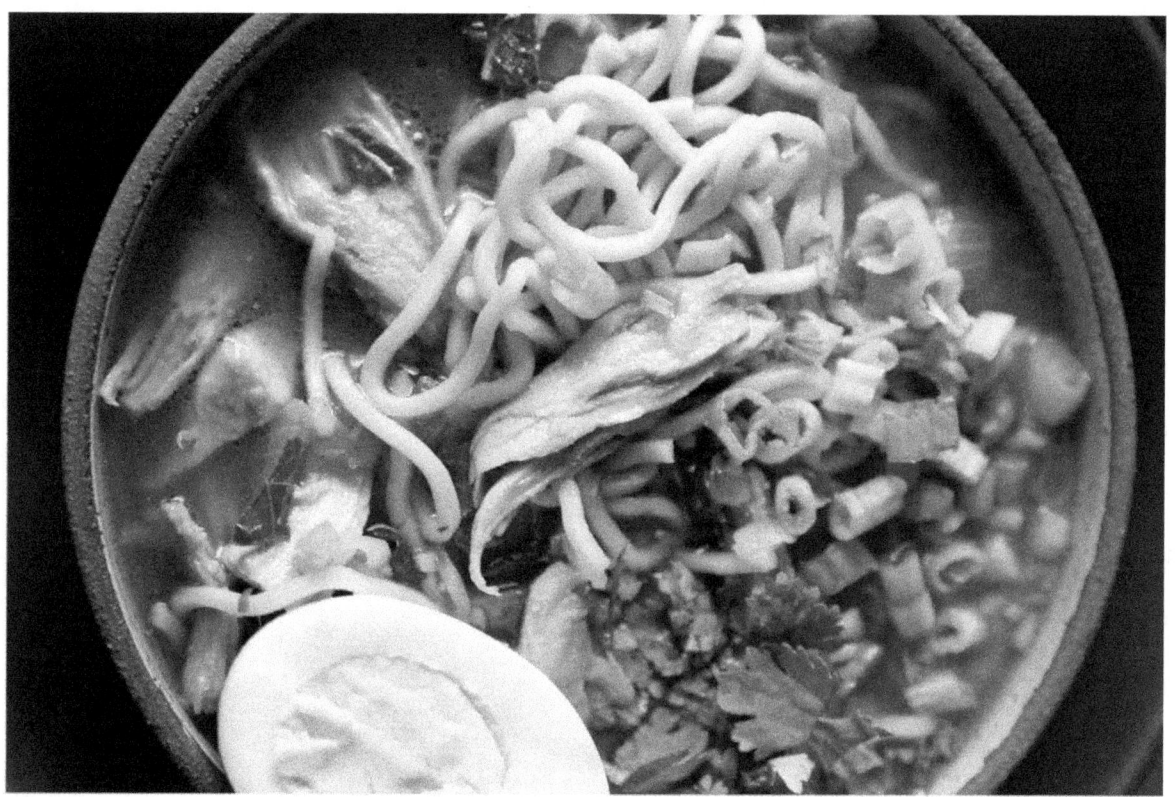

Preparation Time: 10 Minutes

Cooking Time: 20 Minutes

Servings: 2

Ingredients:

One chicken breast

Two eggs

One zucchini, made into noodles

4 cups chicken broth

Two cloves of garlic, peeled and minced

2 tbsps. coconut aminos

3 tbsps. avocado oil

1 tbsp. ginger

Directions:

Pan-fry the chicken in avocado oil in a pan until brown.

Hard boil your eggs and slice them in half.

Add chicken broth to a large pot and simmer with the garlic, coconut aminos, and ginger. Then add in the zucchini noodles for 4-5 mins.

Put the broth into a bowl, top it with eggs and chicken slices, and season to your liking.

Nutrition:

Calories: 478 kcal

Fats: 39 g

Carbs: 3 g

Protein: 31 g

Egg Drop Soup

Eggs are so good in this diet, in our opinion, so there is no better way to finish our recipes than with this great and simple soup.

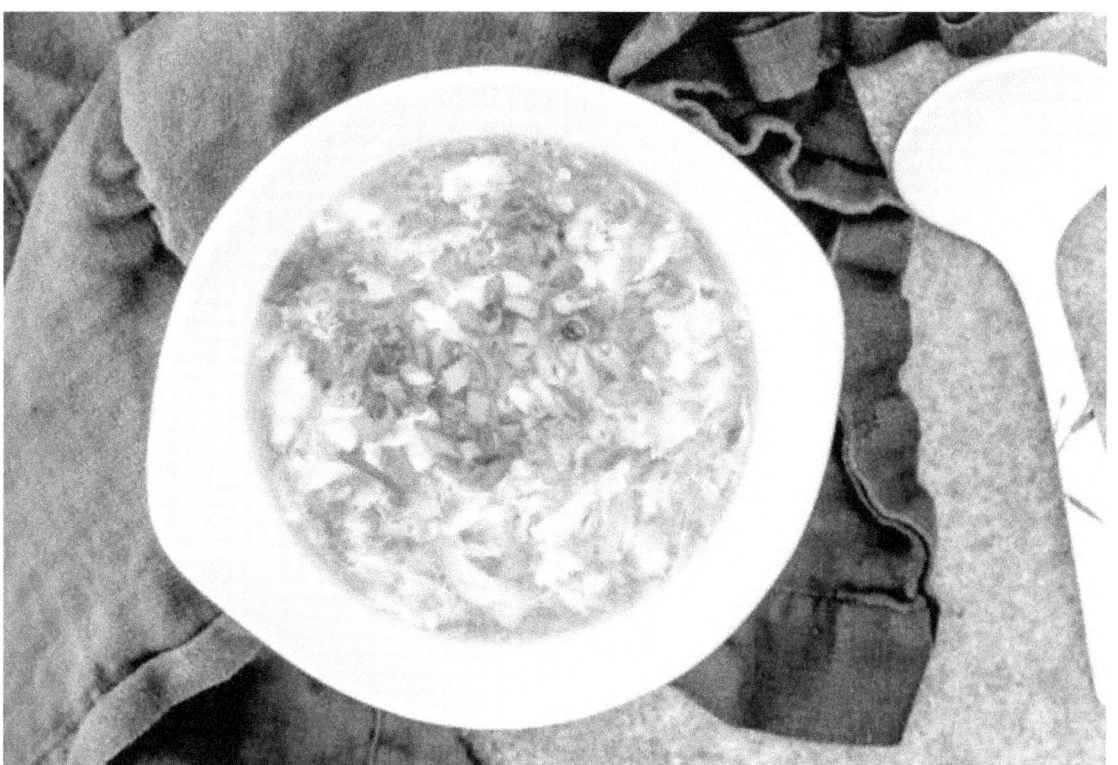

Preparation Time: 5 Minutes

Cooking Time: 15 Minutes

Servings: 2

Ingredients:

3 cups chicken broth

2 cups Swiss chard chopped

Two eggs whisked

1 tsp. grated ginger

1 tsp. ground oregano

2 tbsps. coconut aminos

salt and pepper

Directions:

Heat your broth in a saucepan.

Slowly drizzle in the eggs while stirring slowly.

Add the Swiss chard, grated ginger, oregano, and coconut aminos. Next, season it and let it cook for 5-10 mins.

Nutrition:

Calories: 225 kcal

Fats: 19 g

Carbs: 4 g

Protein: 11 g

CHAPTER 8:

Snack Recipes

1.   Chips

Preparation Time: 10 Minutes

Cooking Time: 20 Minutes

Servings: 4

Ingredients:

You only need five minutes to make this! - You will get four servings from this

Oil spray (make sure its avocado)

 What you need for the coating:

A single tablespoon of paprika - ½ of a tablespoon of cayenne pepper for a little bit of a kick

½ of a tablespoon of onion powder - ¼ of a cup of nutritional yeast - ½ garlic powder

Directions:

What you need for the chip

A bag of pork rinds (take note that whatever bag you choose will change the nutrition information at the end of the recipe)

Add the coating ingredients to a spice grinder and blend until everything becomes smooth.

Spray your pork rinds with oil as it will make the coating stick better.

Transfer the rinds to a plastic bag and pour the toppings in before you begin to shake it.

Nutrition:

Calories-97 - Fat-2.7 grams - Carbs-2 grams - Fiber- 1 gram

Protein-14 grams

Pickle

Preparation Time: 20 Minutes

Cooking Time: 20 Minutes

Servings: 3

Ingredients:

A single can of tuna (go for a version that is light flaked)

¼ of a cup of mayo (it needs to be sugar-free if you can get it and a light version)

A single tablespoon of dill

5 or 6 pickles depending on what you need

Directions:

Cut your pickles in half so that they are lengthwise.

Seed your pickles.

Drain the tuna and then mix the dill, mayo, and tuna in a bowl before mixing.

Spoon the tuna mix onto the pickle.

This will only take you five minutes

You can get up to four servings from this

Nutrition:

A serving size here is based on if you used six pickles.

Another note is that the nutritional information will change depending on what mayo you choose here.

Calories-47.1

Fiber-1.4 grams

Protein 6.01 grams

Carbs- 3.6 grams

Fat-0.6

Hard-boiled eggs

Preparation Time: 20 Minutes

Cooking Time: 20 Minutes

Servings: 12

Ingredients:

A dozen eggs

Directions:

Get a pot that is big enough to hold the eggs.

Place six of the eggs in the pot.

Cover the eggs with cool water by an inch.

Cover your pan with a lid and bring your water to boiling.

Boil water in the pot for six minutes over medium-high heat

If you want them firmer, let them stay in the pot a little longer.

Repeat for the other six.

This is perfect for taking on the go and makes a quick protein-packed snack.

Nutrition:

This is based upon two eggs.

Calories-156

Carbs-1 gram

Fiber-0 grams

Fat-10.6 grams

Protein-12.6 grams

Zingy crackers

Preparation Time: 15 Minutes

Cooking Time: 10 Minutes

Servings: 16

Ingredients:

A single pound cheddar cheese (sliced)

Four sliced jalapeno peppers (use sliced)

Directions:

Heat oven to 425 and then line your baking sheet with parchment

Cut your cheese slices. They need to be 11/2 inch squares.

Arrange them on the baking sheet with at least an inch between them and then place a slice of jalapeno on top.

You will then place them in the oven and bake for a dozen minutes (12).

You will know they are done when they are firm and light brown.

Remove and let them cool.

If stored in an airtight container, they will last two days.

Nutrition:

Calories-106

Protein-7 grams

Carbs-1 gram

Fiber-0.3 grams

Fat-9 grams

Pinwheel Delight

Preparation Time: 5 Minutes

Cooking Time: 5 Minutes

Servings: 20

Ingredients:

A single block of cream cheese (8 ounces)

Ten slices of salami (genoa) and pepperoni

Four tablespoons of pickles (make sure they are finely diced)

Directions:

Have your cream cheese brought to room temperature.

Whip the cream cheese until it becomes fluffy.

Spread your cream cheese in a rectangle that is a quarter-inch thick. Do this on a large piece of plastic wrap.

Place your pickles over cream cheese

Place the salami over the cream cheese in layers that are overlapping so that each cream cheese layer is covered.

Place another layer of the wrap over the layer of salami and press down. Be gentle.

Flip your whole rectangle over so that the bottom cream cheese layer is now facing the top instead.

Peel back your plastic wrap off very carefully from the top cream cheese layer.

You should begin rolling this into a log shape, slowly removing the bottom layer of your plastic wrap as you go along.

Place the pinwheel in a tight plastic wrap.

Place in the fridge overnight or if you can't wait at least four hours.

Slice, however thick you want it.

Nutrition:

Calories- 47 - Fat-4.2 grams - Protein-1 gram - Carbs-0.8 grams

Zesty olives

Preparation Time: 5 Minutes

Cooking Time: 5 Minutes

Servings: 6

Ingredients:

1/4 of a cup of oil (make sure that it is extra virgin olive oil)

1/4 of a teaspoon of pepper flakes (red and crushed) - A single thinly sliced garlic clove

A single tablespoon of lemon juice - A single strip of zest from a lemon

A single cup of olives (make sure that they are castelvetrano)

Two sprigs of thyme (make sure it's fresh)

A single tablespoon of orange juice

A single strip of zest from an orange

Directions:

Get a saucepan.

Heat your oil over medium-high heat.

Add zest, thyme, garlic, and zest in and cook it.

Be sure that you stir occasionally.

Cook for a few minutes, and you will notice that the garlic is golden.

You will then need to stir in the olives and cook them as well.

Stir them as they cook but only cook for two minutes. You want them to be warmed.

Turn off your heat.

Stir in your juice.

Place in a dish.

Nutrition:

Calories-180 - Fat- 20 grams - Carbs- 2 grams

Deviled Eggs Keto Style!

Preparation Time: 5 Minutes

Cooking Time: 5 Minutes

Servings: 20

Ingredients:

Ten eggs (hardboiled of course)

Ten large eggs, hardboiled

A single avocado (make sure it is ripe)

A single lemon (you will need to juice this)

A single tablespoon of mustard (use Dijon)

Paprika (use smoked)

Directions:

Slice your eggs in half and take out the yolks.

Combine your yolks, avocado, and lemon juice in a bowl and stir thoroughly.

Spoon the mixture into the egg halves.

Sprinkle the top with paprika.

Nutrition:

Calories-50

Fat-4 grams

Fiber-1 gram

Protein- 3 grams

Carbs- 1 gram

Cucumber

Preparation Time: 5 Minutes

Cooking Time: 0 Minutes

Servings: 1

Ingredients:

A single cup of cucumbers (make sure they are sliced)

Ten olived (kalamata olives. Use large ones)

Directions:

Mix them in a bowl, and there you go!

Nutrition:

Calories-71

Fiber-2.3 grams

Carbs-5 grams

Fat-4.8 grams

Protein-1.29 grams

Nutty Yogurt

Preparation Time: 5 Minutes

Cooking Time: 0 Minute

Servings: 1

Ingredients:

2 ounces of yogurt (use whole milk greek yogurt)

1/2 of a teaspoon of cinnamon

One tablespoon of walnuts (chopped)

Directions:

Place the yogurt in a dish.

Add the walnuts.

Add the cinnamon.

Nutrition:

Calories-160

Fiber-0.5 grams

Fat-12.5 grams

Protein-8 grams

Carbs-6 grams

Crab

Preparation Time: 5 Minutes

Cooking Time: 5 Minutes

Servings: 4

Ingredients:

A single avocado (make sure that it is ripe)

Three tablespoons of juice from a lemon.

Two tablespoons of chives (chopped)

1/2 of a pound of crab meat (lump)

One teaspoon of mustard (use Dijon)

Directions:

Put your avocados.

Peel them next.

Cut into chunks a half-inch thick.

Place them in a bowl.

Add a tablespoon of your juice.

In a separate bowl, add your other ingredients except for the meat and whisk it together.

Add the meat and toss the ingredients.

Do the same for the last three servings.

Nutrition:

Calories-150

Fat-8 grams

Protein-15 grams

Carbs-5 grams

Fiber-3 grams

Cream And Berries

Preparation Time: 5 Minutes

Cooking Time: 0 Minute

Servings: 1

Ingredients:

A quarter of a cup of berries (raspberries are best)

A single cup of whipping cream

Direction:

Place the whipping cream on the bottom of your bowl.

Place your berries on top.

Nutrition:

Calories-230

Fat-21.5 grams

Protein-2 grams

Fiber- 4 grams

Carbs-5.1 grams

Guacamole

Preparation Time: 5 Minutes

Cooking Time: 5 Minutes

Servings: 1

Ingredients:

Half a cup of guacamole

Half of a cucumber

Directions:

Cut the cucumber into slices after cleaning it.

Serve with the guacamole.

Nutrition:

Calories- 233

Fat-19.9 grams

Fiber-7.7 grams

Carbs-14.9 grams

Protein-3.2 grams

Creamy Dream

Preparation Time: 5 Minutes

Cooking Time: 0 Minutes

Servings: 1

Ingredients:

Two tablespoons almond butter (go with creamy it will mix better)

A single teaspoon of flax seeds

Two teaspoons of pumpkin seeds

A single teaspoon of sunflower seeds

A single teaspoon of chia seeds

Directions:

Get a bowl.

Mix all the ingredients.

The protein that you will get along with the fiber and fat should work to keep you full for longer.

Nutrition:

Calories-262

Fat-21 grams

Carbs-11.6 grams

Protein-11 grams

Fiber-7.8 grams

Creamy Boat

Preparation Time: 5 Minutes

Cooking Time: 0 Minutes

Servings: 4

Ingredients:

Two stalks of celery

Two tablespoons of cream cheese

Directions:

Clean the celery and cut it into pieces.

Place the pieces on a plate before adding cream cheese to them.

Repeat this process if necessary.

Nutrition:

Calories-113

Fat-10.1 grams

Fiber-1.3 grams

Carbs-4 grams

Protein-2.3 grams

CHAPTER 9:

Dessert Recipes

1.   Cheesecake Pumpkin Mousse

Preparation Time: 15 Min

Cooking Time: 0 Min

Serving: 12

Ingredients:

16 ounces cream cheese

15 ounces pumpkin purée

2 cups heavy cream

Two teaspoons pumpkin spice

One teaspoon liquid Stevia

One teaspoon vanilla extract

Directions:

Combine the pumpkin purée with cream cheese in a stand mixer and mix them until they become smooth.

Add in the remaining ingredients and whip them for 5 mins.

Once the time is up, pipe the mousse into serving cups, then serve it and enjoy it.

Nutrition:

Calories: 214

Total Fat: 21 g - Protein: 3.9 g

Total Carbs: 4.2 g

Pumpkin Butter Coffee

Preparation Time: 10 Minutes

Cooking Time: 00 Minutes

Serving: 1

Ingredients:

12 Ounces Hot Brewed Coffee

2 Tablespoons Pumpkin Purée

1 Tablespoon Butter

¼ Teaspoon Pumpkin Spice

Liquid Stevia To Taste

Directions:

Blend Them Smooth.

Serve Your Coffee Right Away And Enjoy.

Nutrition:

Calories: 120 grams

Total Fat: 12 grams

Protein: 1 gram

Total Carbs: 3 grams

Chocolate Pie

Preparation Time: 15 Minutes

Cooking Time: 12 Minutes

Servings: 4

ingredients:

2 cups almond flour

2 cups heavy cream

¼ cup of cocoa powder

Three egg whites

Three tablespoons butter, melted

Three teaspoons Splenda

One teaspoon chilled coffee

1/8 teaspoon liquid Stevia

Salt

Directions:

Preheat the oven to 350 F.

Mix the butter with almond flour, ¼ cup cocoa powder, one teaspoon of Splenda, Stevia, and a pinch of salt in a mixing bowl, then mix them until they become smooth.

Spoon the mix into a baking pan to make the crust and bake it for 12 mins, then set it aside to cool down.

Beat the egg whites with 2/3 cup of cocoa powder, two teaspoons of Splenda, coffee, heavy cream, and a pinch of salt in a large bowl until they become fluffy and light to make the filling.

Pour the filling into the crust, bake it, then chill it in the fridge for 2 hours, then serve it and enjoy it.

Nutrition:

Calories: 630 - Total Fat: 57.2 g - Protein: 17.6 g - Total Carbs: 26 g

Chocolate Mousse

Preparation Time: 15 Minutes

Cooking Time: 00 Minutes

Servings: 4

Ingredients:

8.5 ounces mascarpone cheese

Two tablespoons cocoa powder, unsweetened

One tablespoon of a sweetener

One teaspoon vanilla extract

Directions:

Spoon the mousse into serving cups, then serve them and enjoy.

Nutrition:

Calories: 286

Total Fat: 27 g

Protein: 4 g

Total Carbs: 2 g

Pomegranate Pudding

Preparation Time: 15 Minutes

Cooking Time: 10 Minutes

Servings: 4

Ingredients:

14.5 ounces coconut milk

½ cup pomegranate seeds

Three tablespoons raw honey

Two tablespoons coconut oil

One tablespoon vanilla extract

One packet gelatin, unflavored

Directions:

Stir in the honey with coconut milk and vanilla extract.

Cook the coconut mix until it starts bubbling, then stir in the gelatin gently until it completely melts.

Stir in the pomegranate seeds and pour the mixture into serving cups, then refrigerate them for 4 hours.

Serve the coconut pudding and enjoy it.

Nutrition:

Calories: 386

Total Fat: 31.3 g

Protein: 8.6 g

Total Carbs: 21.5 g

Berry Lemon Cake

Preparation Time: 15 Min

Cooking Time: 30 Minutes

Serving: 6

Ingredients:

½ cup fresh blueberries

½ cup coconut flour

1/3 cup coconut milk

1/3 cup raw honey

Three eggs, beaten

2 ½ tablespoons coconut oil, melted

Two tablespoons fresh lemon juice

One tablespoon lemon zest, grated

One teaspoon lemon extract

One teaspoon apple cider vinegar

½ teaspoon baking soda

Salt

Directions:

Preheat the oven to 350 F.

Mix the apple cider with baking soda in a small bowl.

Mix the baking soda mix with coconut oil, lemon juice, and zest, lemon extract, coconut flour and honey, coconut milk, eggs, and a pinch of salt until no lumps are found, then fold in the berries.

Pour the batter into a greased baking dish, then bake it for 30 mins.

Nutrition:

Calories: 203 - Total Fat: 13.4 g - Protein: 3.5 g - Total Carbs: 19.6 g

Vanilla Cupcakes

Preparation Time: 15 Minutes

Cooking Time: 30 Minutes

Servings: 32

Ingredients:

1 cup almond milk, unsweetened

1 cup almond flour

¾ cup erythritol, powdered

½ cup butter

Seven eggs

One tablespoon baking powder

Three teaspoons vanilla extract

½ teaspoon liquid stevia

Salt

Directions:

Preheat the oven to 350 F.

Pour the batter into cupcake liners, then bake them for 28 to 30 mins.

Allow the cupcakes to cool, then serve them with your favorite toppings and enjoy.

Nutrition:

Calories: 100

Total Fat: 7.1 g

Protein: 2.1 g

Total Carbs: 8 g

Cocoa Mocha Truffles

Preparation Time: 15 Minutes

Cooking Time: 00 Minutes

Servings: 15 To 20

Ingredients:

7 ounces butter, unsalted

Four tablespoons strong brewed coffee

Two tablespoons honey

Two tablespoons cocoa powder

½ teaspoon vanilla powder

½ teaspoon cinnamon

Salt

Directions:

Spoon two teaspoons of the mix and shape it into balls, then roll them in some cocoa powder or chopped nuts.

Repeat the process with the remaining mix, freeze them for 1 hour, then serve them and enjoy.

Nutrition:

Calories: 93

Total Fat: 9.6 g

Protein: 0.2 g

Total Carbs: 2.5 g

Vanilla Ice Cream

Preparation Time: 20 Minutes

Cooking Time: 00 Minutes

Servings: 6

Ingredients:

Four egg whites

Four egg yolks

One ¼ cup heavy whipping cream

½ cup erythritol, powdered

One tablespoon vanilla extract

¼ teaspoon cream of tartar

Directions:

Whisk the whipped cream in another bowl until it's soft peaks.

Whisk the egg yolks until they become pale, then add the vanilla and whisk them again.

Spoon the mix into a loaf pan and freeze it for 2 hours, then serve your ice cream and enjoy it.

Nutrition:

Calories: 226

Total Fat: 12.3 g

Protein: 4.8 g

Total Carbs: 24.9 g

Snow Bites

Preparation Time: 20 Minutes

Cooking Time: 18 Minutes

Servings: 36

Ingredients:

2 cups almond flour - 1 cup walnuts, finely chopped - ¾ and ½ cup erythritol, powdered

½ cup butter softened - One egg - Two tablespoons coconut flour

One teaspoon vanilla extract - One teaspoon baking powder

¾ teaspoon cardamom powder

¼ teaspoon Stevia extract

Salt

Directions:

Preheat the oven to 325 F.

Mix the cardamom powder with a pinch of salt, coconut flour, walnut, baking powder, and almond flour in a mixing bowl.

Beat ½ cup of erythritol with butter in a mixing bowl until it becomes light and fluffy, then add the egg with Stevia and vanilla and beat them again.

Add the almond mix to the butter and mix them until they make a smooth dough, then shape it into ¾ inch balls.

Place the dough balls on two lined baking sheets and bake them for 18 mins.

Once the time is up, toss the almond balls in a large bowl gently with ¾ cup of erythritol until coated, then serve them and enjoy.

Nutrition:

Calories: 40 - Total Fat: 7.4 g

Protein: 2.1 g - Total Carbs: 5.5 g

Blueberry Ice Cream

Preparation Time: 15 Minutes

Cooking Time: 00 Minutes

Servings: 4

Ingredients:

1 cup heavy whipping cream

½ cup crème Fraiche

½ cup blueberries

Two egg yolks

One tablespoon vanilla powder

Directions:

Whip the whipping cream until it becomes fluffy, then set it aside.

Beat the crème Fraiche until it becomes fluffy, then add the whipping cream, vanilla, blueberries, and egg yolks and beat them again until they become creamy.

Spoon the ice cream into a loaf pan and freeze it for 1 hour, then serve it and enjoy it.

Nutrition:

Calories: 202

Total Fat: 19 g

Protein: 2.4 g

Total Carbs: 4.6 g

Pecan Pie Ice Cream

Preparation Time: 15 Minutes

Cooking Time: 00 Minutes

Servings: 4

Ingredients:

2 cups of coconut milk

½ cup pumpkin purée

½ cup cottage cheese

½ cup pecans, toasted and chopped

1/3 cup erythritol, powdered

Three egg yolks

20 drops liquid Stevia

One teaspoon pumpkin spice

One teaspoon maple extract

½ teaspoon xanthan gum powder

Directions:

blend them with an immersion blender until they become smooth.

2. Pour the mix into an ice cream machine and stir in the toasted pecans, then Preparation it according to the manufacturer's instructions.

Serve your ice cream and enjoy it.

Nutrition:

Calories: 467

Total Fat: 37.2 g

Protein: 6 g

Total Carbs: 34.3 g

Chocolate Bites

Preparation Time: 20 Minutes

Cooking Time: 20 Minutes

Servings: 20

Ingredients:

1 cup almond flour

1/3 cup coconut, shredded

1/3 cup erythritol, powdered

¼ cup of coconut oil

¼ cup of cocoa powder

Two eggs

Three tablespoons coconut flour

One teaspoon vanilla extract

½ teaspoon baking powder

Salt

Directions:

Preheat the oven to 350 F.

Mix the shredded coconut and coconut flour with cocoa powder, erythritol, almond flour, baking powder, and a pinch of salt in a large bowl.

Add the vanilla with coconut oil and eggs, then knead them to get a smooth dough.

Shape the dough into 20 balls, then place them on a lined baking sheet and bake them for 15 to 20 mins.

Once the time is up, serve your chocolate bites and enjoy it.

Nutrition:

Calories: 85 - Total Fat: 6.4 g - Protein: 1.9 g - Total Carbs: 6.7 g

Swiss Roll

Preparation Time: 25 Minutes

Cooking Time: 15 Minutes

Servings:12

Ingredients:

8 ounces cream cheese - 1 cup almond flour - ½ cup erythritol, powder - ½ cup sour cream

¼ cup of cocoa powder - ¼ cup of coconut milk - ¼ cup psyllium husk powder

12 tablespoons butter - Three eggs - Two teaspoons vanilla extract

One teaspoon baking powder

¼ teaspoon liquid Stevia

Salt

Directions:

Mix the almond flour with ¼ cup of cocoa powder, psyllium husk powder, baking powder, ¼ cup of erythritol, and a pinch of salt in a large mixing bowl.

Add in 4 tablespoons of butter with coconut milk, ¼ cup of sour cream, eggs, and one teaspoon of vanilla extract and mix them again until they become smooth.

Preheat the oven to 350 F.

Transfer the mix to a lined baking sheet and press it to make the crust, then bake it for 12 to 15 mins.

Beat the remaining eight tablespoons of butter with ¼ cup of erythritol, one teaspoon of vanilla, Stevia, ¼ cup of sour cream, and cream cheese until they become light and fluffy to make the filling.

Spread the filling all over the crust and roll it gently.

Serve your Swiss Roll with your favorite toppings and enjoy.

Nutrition:

Calories: 274.2 - Total Fat: 25.1 g - Protein: 5.3 g - Total Carbs: 6.8 g

CHAPTER 10:

30 Days Meal Plan

Each of these recipes has the net carbs per serving posted. You will see how flexible the plan is when you look at how easy it is to use just the recipes in this cookbook for 30 full days, including three meals, snacks, and desserts.

The meals are planned, so you still have flexibility in your eating patterns with extra carbs to use as desired. Even on the strictest diet plan, most of these recipes should be just what the doctor ordered. Calculate how many carbs you are allowed each day and add some healthy snacks or sides to these totals. It's all up to you; just track everything.

Days	Breakfast	Lunch	Dinner	Dessert/Snack
Day 1	Peanut Butter Chocolate Protein Shake Or Roasted Brussels Sprouts Salad With Parmesan	Pork Cutlets with Spanish Onion And Roasted Brussels Sprouts Salad With Parmesan	Roasted Brussels Sprouts Salad With Parmesan	Chips And Cheesecake Pumpkin Mousse
Day 2	Creamy Dreamy Green Smoothie Or Roasted Brussels Sprouts Salad With Parmesan	Rich and Easy Pork Ragout And Blue Cheese And Bacon Kale Salad	Wedge Salad and Creamy Broccoli and Leek Soup	Pickle And Pumpkin Butter Coffee

Day 3	Blueberry-Flax Yogurt Parfait Or Wedge Salad	Melt-in-Your-Mouth Pork Roast Or Mom's Festive Meatloaf	Mexican Egg Salad And Chicken Soup	Hard-boiled eggs And Chocolate Pie
Day 4	Salted Peanut Butter and Chocolate Yogurt Cup Or Mexican Egg Salad	Chunky Pork Soup with Mustard Greens Or Chopped Greek Salad	Blue Cheese And Bacon Kale Salad And Greek Egg and Lemon Soup with Chicken	Zingy crackers And Chocolate Mousse
Day 5	Crunchy Nut and Seed Granola Or Blue Cheese And Bacon Kale Salad	Pulled Pork with Mint and Cheese	Chopped Greek Salad And Zucchini Cream Soup	Pinwheel Delight And Pomegranate Pudding
Day 6	Classic Pancakes Or Chopped Greek Salad	Pork Loin Steaks in Creamy Pepper Sauce And	Mediterranean Cucumber Salad And	Zesty olives And Berry Lemon Cake

		Mediterranean Cucumber Salad	Cauli Soup	
Day 7	Orange Ricotta–Stuffed Crêpes Or Mediterranean Cucumber Salad	Pork Medallions with Cabbage And Avocado Egg Salad Lettuce Cups	Avocado Egg Salad Lettuce Cups And Keto Fish	Deviled Eggs Keto Style! And Vanilla Cupcakes
Day 8	Cauliflower Hash Browns Or Avocado Egg Salad Lettuce Cups	Mom's Festive Meatloaf	Roasted Brussels Sprouts Salad With Parmesan And Zingy Lemon Fish	Cucumber And Cocoa Mocha Truffles
Day 9	Creamy Broccoli and Leek Soup And Pickle	Rich Winter Beef Stew	Wedge Salad And Creamy Keto Fish Casserole	Nutty Yogurt And Vanilla Ice Cream
Day 10	Chicken Soup And Cheesecake Pumpkin Mousse	Mini Meatloaves with Spinach And Keto Fish Casserole With	Mexican Egg Salad	Crab And Snow Bites

		Mushrooms And French Mustard		
Day 11	Greek Egg and Lemon Soup with Chicken	Keto Fish Or Keto Thai Fish With Curry And Coconut	Blue Cheese And Bacon Kale Salad	Cream And Berries And Blueberry Ice Cream
Day 12	Wild Mushroom Soup	Zingy Lemon Fish	Chopped Greek Salad	Guacamole And Pecan Pie Ice Cream
Day 13	Zucchini Cream Soup	Creamy Keto Fish Casserole	Mediterranean Cucumber Salad	Creamy Dream And Swiss Roll
Day 14	Cauli Soup	Keto Fish Casserole With Mushrooms And French Mustard	Avocado Egg Salad Lettuce Cups	Creamy boat And Chocolate Bites
Day 15	Thai Coconut Soup	Keto Thai Fish With Curry And Coconut	Roasted Brussels Sprouts Salad With Parmesan	Cheesecake Pumpkin Mousse Or

				Cocoa Mocha Truffles
Day 16	Chicken Ramen Soup	Pork Cutlets with Spanish Onion	Wedge Salad	Pumpkin Butter Coffee Or Vanilla Cupcakes
Day 17	Egg Drop Soup	Rich and Easy Pork Ragout	Mexican Egg Salad	Chocolate Pie Or Berry Lemon Cake
Day 18	Peanut Butter Chocolate Protein Shake	Melt-in-Your-Mouth Pork Roast	Blue Cheese And Bacon Kale Salad	Chocolate Mousse And Pomegranate Pudding
Day 19	Creamy Dreamy Green Smoothie	Chunky Pork Soup with Mustard Greens And Keto Fish Casserole With	Chopped Greek Salad	Pomegranate Pudding And Chocolate Mousse

		Mushrooms And French Mustard		
Day 20	Blueberry-Flax Yogurt Parfait	Pulled Pork with Mint and Cheese And Blue Cheese And Bacon Kale Salad	Mediterranean Cucumber Salad	Berry Lemon Cake And Chocolate Pie
Day 21	Salted Peanut Butter and Chocolate Yogurt Cup	Pork Loin Steaks in Creamy Pepper Sauce And Mediterranean Cucumber Salad	Avocado Egg Salad Lettuce Cups	Vanilla Cupcakes And Pumpkin Butter Coffee
Day 22	Crunchy Nut and Seed Granola	Pork Medallions with Cabbage And Avocado Egg Salad Lettuce Cups	Roasted Brussels Sprouts Salad With Parmesan	Cocoa Mocha Truffles
Day 23	Classic Pancakes	Mom's Festive Meatloaf And	Wedge Salad	Vanilla Ice Cream And

		Creamy Broccoli and Leek Soup		Cheesecake Pumpkin Mousse
Day 24	Orange Ricotta–Stuffed Crêpes	Rich Winter Beef Stew And Creamy Broccoli and Leek Soup	Mexican Egg Salad	Snow Bites And Deviled Eggs Keto Style!
Day 25	Cauliflower Hash Browns	Mini Meatloaves with Spinach And Creamy Broccoli and Leek Soup	Blue Cheese And Bacon Kale Salad	Blueberry Ice Cream And Zesty olives
Day 26	Creamy Broccoli and Leek Soup	Keto Fish And Greek Egg and Lemon Soup with Chicken	Chopped Greek Salad	Pecan Pie Ice Cream And Pinwheel Delight
Day 27	Chicken Soup	Zingy Lemon Fish And Greek Egg and Lemon Soup with Chicken	Mediterranean Cucumber Salad	Chocolate Bites And Zingy crackers

Day 28	Greek Egg and Lemon Soup with Chicken	Creamy Keto Fish Casserole And Greek Egg and Lemon Soup with Chicken	Avocado Egg Salad Lettuce Cups	Swiss Roll And Hard-boiled eggs
Day 29	Wild Mushroom Soup	Keto Fish Casserole With Mushrooms And French Mustard	Roasted Brussels Sprouts Salad With Parmesan And Keto Thai Fish With Curry And Coconut	Pinwheel Delight And Pickle
Day 30	Zucchini Cream Soup	Keto Thai Fish With Curry And Coconut	Wedge Salad And Keto Fish Casserole With Mushrooms And French Mustard	Guacamole And Chips

CHAPTER 11:

How to Start a Keto Diet After 50

Trying to lose weight can be intimidating at any age. However, once you're in your fifties, it becomes even more overwhelming. Most of us know this happens, but only a few know why. After the age of 25, which is when the body stops bone growth, the metabolic rate goes down by about 2% over every ten years. So the number of calories you can consume without gaining weight also decreases by each decade. This is why it is important to increase your levels of activity, as well as be more conscious of your food intake.

As you grow older, it becomes more difficult to lose weight as easily as, say, five years before, and due to this, most people lose hope of dropping weight as they grow.

Here are a few ways you can start your keto diet:

Set A Date

Planning a date to start your Keto journey doesn't necessarily mean you need a date to go shopping or meal prepping. It means that you will prepare yourself mentally for the change in your lifestyle. This also means letting your loved ones know that you will soon embark on this journey that may or may not be easy and that you will need their support and encouragement. Informing people around you about your lifestyle change encourages them to be more thoughtful and considerate about your dietary restrictions, and they might create dinner or lunch plans with you according to your new lifestyle.

Create A Routine

Adopting a good routine, especially in the morning, can help you in your journey. Start your day by drinking plenty of water and consuming a teaspoon of coconut oil. Make sure that you get a good night's sleep, and stay active during the day, as well as taking some time out daily to exercise.

Get Rid of Non-Keto Foods

Most of us are guilty of indulging in unhealthy foods a few days before we embark on this journey of ketogenic weight loss. To avoid this from happening, throw away all and any non-ketogenic foods from your food cabinets and refrigerator. A mistake that most of us make when starting a healthier diet is to think that the motivation of losing weight will be the same throughout, and you won't be tempted to eat that chocolate bar lying around in your refrigerator. However, adopting a healthy lifestyle and being consistent can be challenging, so to not risk indulging in guilty pleasures, it is best to get rid of all non-keto foods from your life and home.

Try Intermittent Fasting

Intermittent fasting is considered to be a foolproof way to control your intake of carbohydrates adequately. Intermittent fasting may seem scary to most people, as we talk about a certain number of hours without consuming foods. A great way to go about it without letting it seem too daunting, and instead of counting hours, you just have to skip one meal every day. Most doctors suggest having a late breakfast or brunch, and an early dinner later on. This automatically creates a fast of 12 to 13 hours.

Consume Less Than 25 Grams of Carbs Daily

To get your body to transition to ketosis and for it to be motivated into burning fat, you need to increase your intake of healthy fats and lower your intake of carbohydrates. It is recommended to keep your carbohydrate consumption to less than 25 grams a day. Start leaning towards healthy fats and proteins, such as coconut oil, avocados, and eggs. When the body gets more of fats and fewer carbs, it has a good balance, and there isn't a lack of ketones.

Counting Carbs for Beginners

Perhaps the most impressive aspect of keto is learning how to control your carbs. But here's the thing, you may have some limitations when you're only a beginner. In the beginning, stick to a total of 20 grams of net carbs each day. We have explained how to calculate net carbs in the later (net carbs are the carbohydrate which is absorbed). This milestone is usually the starting point for most people as they start keto for the first time.

We urge you to stick to these guidelines and follow them for at least three months. For the keto diet to work, you'll need to make sure your body's going through ketosis. One of the most reliable ways to test this is by regularly checking your blood with a blood ketone testing meter. (If you're planning on switching to keto for the long run, this is an investment worth making).

Your blood ketone levels should rise to 0.1 mmol/L when you're new to the diet. 0.5 mmol/L is the stage that indicates that you're in ketosis now.

The good old keto flu is another sign that indicates the diet is working.

What is Your Carbs Limit?

This is the minimal amount of carbs you can consume without kicking out your body from the state of ketosis.

Factors That May Affect Your Daily Carb Limit

Now here's the thing, your daily carb limit isn't set to stone and can be influenced by a whole bunch of factors. Here are some factors which you might need to take into account:

Emotional Stress

Emotional stress can alter insulin response and a whole bunch of stress hormones. So your blood glucose level might be particularly high on a stressful day. This will get on the way of the ketone on your body. To maintain a healthy lifestyle, practice ways to manage stress, you can go for a long walk, or talk to a friend. Learning how to manage stress is an excellent way to take care of your overall well-being.

Exercising and Heavy Workouts

Exercise, particularly long and tedious workouts, can influence your glucose levels in many ways. Performing intense workouts without taking breaks can raise cortisol levels that also impact glucose and ends up increasing its levels in the blood. This is why it is important to rest and allow your body enough time to recover.

Also, you might experience a sudden spike in glucose levels after working out. This is normal and will tend to subside after an hour or so. That being said, seniors are better off practicing lightweight exercises, which will not only burn more fats but will help you reach ketosis much faster.

Coffee can also affect insulin levels in the body. For instance, some people might experience a spike in glucose levels, while others may find that coffee helps with insulin sensitivity. If you're a fan of caffeine, we suggest you test your glucose levels 30 minutes before having a cup and 30 minutes after.

Sleep Cycle

Research conducted by Cedars-Sinai Medical Center in Los Angeles, CA, has indicated how sleep deprivation is known to hamper fasting insulin sensitivity. So, if you're not getting enough sleep, you might experience a change in your blood glucose levels. If you're interested in testing out this hypothesis, simply check your blood glucose levels with a full night's sleep and once when your sleep's been interrupted.

Understanding How to Calculate Net Carbs

If you're new to the whole keto frenzy, then you're probably wondering how you should calculate your carbs. Before we get down to the specifics, it's important to understand what net carbs are. This is a term that you are likely to come across when looking at food nutrition labels. When browsing true nutrition labels, you will find substances such as sugar, alcohol, and fiber under the carbohydrate category.

To find out your daily carb count, you will need to keep track of the net carbs that you are consuming. It's important to understand here that not all types of carbohydrates such as insoluble fiber spike up blood sugar levels; hence you don't have to keep track of these substances when counting carbs.

How to Calculate Net Carbs?

One simple way to calculate the number of net carbs in whole foods is to content from the total number of carbohydrates. When calculating net carbs for processed foods, you'll have to subtract the number of fiber and sugar alcohols from total carbs.

Fiber: Though fiber is a type of carbohydrate found in plants, your body doesn't have the enzyme to digest it. Hence, the fiber content you consume is digested without any change. Simply subtract out the fiber content from the total carbohydrates count, and you're good to go.

Sugar alcohols: While sugar alcohols such as erythritol and xylitol taste sweet, they are only partially digested by the body and largely remain indigestible. Hence when buying food, you can quickly subtract the sugar alcohol content from the total number of carbohydrates.

However, it's important to note that not all sugar alcohols are completely carb-free. Here's where you'll need to be wary of manufacturers who forcefully try to make their products seem lower carb then they are.

You can easily combat this problem by being aware of the different types of sugar alcohol. Xylitol, erythritol, lactitol, and mannitol are sugar alcohols that you don't have to count when calculating net carbs.

On the other hand, maltitol, isomalt, glycerin, and sorbitol count as about half a gram carb. When counting these sugar alcohols, all you have to do is take the total number of grams and divide it by 2.

A simple way to depict this equation is through the following:

Net carbs = total carbs – fiber – sugar alcohols + (maltitol, isomalt, glycerin and sorbitol/ 2)

It is important to calculate these carbs as Keto requires you to keep count of every single gram of carbohydrate you consume.

The Ultimate Keto Shopping List

Here's where you start your keto journey. It's time you go shopping. Here's a list of essential keto items you should include in your shopping list:

Foods to Eat

We all know that a ketogenic diet is based on eating healthy fats and lowering the carbs. However, it isn't as simple as this. Here are the foods that are your best friends in a keto diet:

Meat: Meat is a keto-friendly food; however, it should be unprocessed. Named meat for a keto diet would be organic. As meat is a great source of protein, and keto is based on a high-fat diet, meat is a portion of free food that doesn't need to be consumed in high amounts.

Seafood: Seafood, and especially fatty fish, including salmon, is good to consume when following a keto diet. You can grill the seafood or cook it without breading.

Eggs: Eggs are the most popular food on the keto menu. You can have them in any way you prefer, from boiled to scrambled or even as an omelet. As healthy fats are good in this diet, making eggs in butter will become a treat. Similar to meat, try to look for organic eggs.

Natural fat: As keto diet consists of mainly consuming fats, you can use oils like coconut oil and olive oil to cook your food in.

Vegetables: Consuming vegetables in any diet is always beneficial. In a keto diet, eat vegetables that are above grown, as they are mostly low in carbs. Root vegetables mostly contain a higher number of carbs and should be consumed sparingly.

High-fat dairy: Dairy food like butter, cheese, and heavy creams are all a yes in the ketogenic diet and, is one of the reasons why it is so popular amongst dairy lovers.

Nuts: Many people think that nuts can be consumed as much as one wants in the keto diet. However, nuts can be eaten in a moderate amount as nuts like cashews are high in carbohydrates.

Berries: One of the most popular keto desserts are berries topped with whipped cream. However, like nuts, berries should be consumed in moderation.

Avocados: Avocados are loved by everyone on a keto diet. They are healthy and delicious and come with many health benefits.

CHAPTER 12:

The Ketogenic Diet Rules

I n this, we'll explore the rules of eating keto. You'll learn the how's and whys of keto living, especially as it pertains to the goal of getting 70 percent of your calories from fat, 20 percent from protein, and 10 percent from carbohydrates. I'll also throw in some special tips and tricks that will make the job easier.

Eat Mostly Fat

The keto diet operates by restricting carbohydrates and encouraging the consumption of high amounts of fat. The goal is to reach a state of ketosis, where your body burns fat for energy due to the lack of carbohydrates. To achieve this, you'll want to set a daily goal that 70 to 75 percent of your calories come from fat.

The easiest way to reach your daily goal is to incorporate foods into your diet that have macros of 75 percent fat or higher. Some keto-friendly (and tasty) things you're probably already eating, along With Their Fat Percentages, Are:

Butter, 100%

Mayonnaise, 100%

Heavy Whipping Cream, 95%

Sour Cream, 93%

Ranch Dressing, 93%

Macadamia Nuts, 90%

Cream Cheese, 87%

Bacon, 85%

Pork Sausage, 80%

Egg Yolks, 79%

Salmon, 76%

Avocados, 75%

In 1950, physiologist Dr. Ancel Keys hypothesized that saturated fat caused cardiovascular heart disease and should be avoided. In many studies, since this hypothesis has been debunked. Some fats are healthier than others, but whether it's unsaturated fats found in foods like avocados, nuts, and olive oils, or saturated fats found in foods like butter, red meat, and eggs, they're all beneficial in some way.

There are some unhealthy fat sources to stay away from, including processed trans fats and vegetable oils (oils extracted from seeds), such as corn, canola, grapeseed, peanut, soybean, and sunflower oils, margarine, and vegetable shortening.

Moderate Protein Intake

Protein balance is important. Generally, your goal in keto is to keep protein around 20 to 25 percent of your total calories. The body converts excess protein into glucose, a process called gluconeogenesis, which can potentially kick you out of ketosis. However, protein does a great job of keeping you full, so you don't want to eat too little, either. If you find yourself getting hungry, a little protein will usually do the trick.

Unlike fats and carbs, protein isn't stored in the body, so it's important to get enough protein every day. Protein is essential for strong bones and building a healthy immune system. A protein deficiency can cause hair loss, skin problems, nail issues, and even result in muscle loss, as well as put you at an increased risk of illness.

Generally, I would recommend following the guideline of getting 20 to 25 percent of your daily calories from protein, but people react differently to protein. If you eat more than that and you're having an issue staying in ketosis, simply drop back a little. The important thing is to make sure you always get enough protein.A great way to stay in balance with fat and protein is to eat fattier cuts of meat. Some good choices include a beef ribeye or New York strip steak, chicken thighs, pork ribs, and hamburger meat—all easily ordered in a restaurant or thrown on the grill at home. Lean meats like skinless chicken, turkey, beef, and pork that have been trimmed of fat are fine as well, but you'll need to compensate with fat elsewhere to meet your goal.

Restrict Carbohydrates

You've learned that to reach ketosis and start burning fat as fuel, you must dramatically restrict your carb intake. Everyone is different, but generally, you should be eating around 30 to 50 carbs per day, which will work out to around 5 to 10 percent of your calories. Some people may be able to eat additional carbs and stay in ketosis, while others might need to cut back.

Keto is a pretty restrictive lifestyle concerning carbs, and some people find it easier to start by staying under 20 net carbs per day instead of tracking macros or percentages. I did this in the beginning, and it worked well for me. For the first few months, I aimed for 20 net carbs daily, and anything that fits in that calculation was fair game. I was able to lose 15 pounds quickly, and during that time, I became very familiar with the different carb counts on food items and how they affected my ability to reach and stay in ketosis. When my weight loss began to slow down and stall, I started tracking macros. It was a smooth transition, and I began to lose weight once again.

Net Carbs

You can track either total carbs or net carbs. Total carbs mean all the carbs that a serving of food contains. Net carbs are the actual carbs absorbed by the body that have an impact on your blood sugar. To calculate the net carbs of whole food, such as a piece of fruit, we take the total amount of carbs minus fiber. For example, an avocado has 16 grams of carbs and 12 grams of fiber. So, 16 - 12 = 4 net carbs. Fiber doesn't get used in the body because it doesn't break down, so it can be deducted.

Sugar Alcohols

Sugar alcohols are human-made sweeteners used in many low-carb goodies, and we'll use some of them in recipes in this book. Examples are erythritol, maltitol, sorbitol, and xylitol. Some can be substituted directly for sugar, and some are much sweeter. Sugar alcohols operate a lot like fiber in that they don't get used in the body because they don't break down, so they can also be deducted to determine net carbs. The equation is carbs - fiber - sugar alcohols = net carbs.

Not all sugar alcohols are created equal, however, and not everyone can achieve and stay in ketosis while eating them. There are the lucky few who can down any goody with sugar alcohols and see no effect on their level of ketosis, and others who can eat the same thing and get thrown out. It's simply a trial-and-error process.

Hydrate, Hydrate, Hydrate

Dehydration is a common side effect of ketosis. Your body is used to eating carbs and storing that energy as glycogen (the stored form of glucose). When you restrict carbs and burn through all your stored glucose, you lose a great deal of water weight and electrolytes in the process. High levels of ketones can also cause frequent urination, further contributing to the loss of water and electrolytes.

When starting a keto diet, this loss of water weight and electrolytes can make you feel run-down and nauseated, and something described earlier as the keto flu. It's crucial from the very start, and throughout ketosis, to always stay hydrated; otherwise, you may experience headaches, muscle cramps and spasms, weakness, fatigue, and more.

The simple way to treat and avoid dehydration is by drinking more water, electrolyte supplements, sugar-free electrolyte sports drinks, pickle juice, bone broth, and consuming more liquids in general.

Bulletproof Coffee

Bulletproof coffee, BPC for short, is a delicious, high-fat, high-calorie concoction that's used to enhance energy and endurance before a workout. The original recipe came from Dave Asprey, the creator of the Bulletproof Diet. It also serves as a substitute for breakfast or a quick "pick-me-up" throughout the day. BPC is made with 8 to 12 ounces of freshly brewed coffee, 1 to 2 tablespoons of unsalted butter, whipping cream or half-and-half, and 1 to 2 tablespoons of medium-chain triglyceride (MCT) coconut oil or powder. MCT oil can be a little hard on your stomach, so some people prefer the powder. Some people also add collagen powder, artificial sweeteners, unsweetened cocoa, or other sugar-free flavors. I like to add Perfect Keto's MCT oil powder and their collagen powder to mine. You can use a frothier or blender to turn BPC into a creamy latte, or simply stir it up. BPC is considered great for keto, as the high-fat butter keeps you satiated and full for hours, while the MCT oil or powder provides quick, clean energy and aids in appetite suppression—all via hot, caffeinated coffee.

What About Intermittent Fasting?

Intermittent fasting involves eating within a window of 8 hours and fasting for the remaining 16, a method that can provide benefits in the keto lifestyle. A sample eating window for someone doing intermittent fasting might start with the first meal of the day at 11:00 a.m. and end with the final meal of the day eight hours later at 7:00 p.m. The rest of the day, from after your last meal at 7:00 p.m. until your first meal the next day at 11:00 a.m., is spent fasting. Some people shorten their eating windows to between four and six hours, but eight is fine.

When combined, keto and intermittent fasting yield outstanding results. Keto mimics fasting in that it forces the body to burn fat for energy when starved of carbohydrates. Intermittent fasting sets the body up to efficiently burn fat between meals by lowering insulin, which can be very helpful to reach and stay in ketosis or achieve more aggressive weight-loss results.

The eight-hour eating window can be altered to fit any schedule, but it's best to eat earlier in the day and not snack at all, especially at night, although you'll want to stay hydrated at all times. Studies have shown that eating early and fasting at night also helps with metabolism. It's not for everyone and certainly not mandatory—just another method worth considering as you explore the keto lifestyle.

CHAPTER 13:

Low Carb, High Fat, All Natural

The ketogenic (keto) diet is a low-carb, high-fat diet that makes losing weight simple. It's important to balance the low-carbs with a high fat intake, which can seem a little counterintuitive if, like so many of us, you've grown up being told that fat makes you fat. But it's high-quality fats such as coconut oil, avocado, and butter from grass-fed cows that fuel your body once you enter ketosis— so fat is an incredibly important piece of the keto puzzle.

Ketosis is what makes keto work, so you should know that it's essentially the metabolic process in which the body stops using glucose (sugar) for energy and burns fats instead. Getting into ketosis involves more than just estimating and trying to eat as low-carb as possible, so do use a keto calculator online and enter your height, weight, estimated body fat percentage, and weight-loss goals. A calculator will give you a daily calorie count and your carb, fat, and protein macros. If you follow the guidelines, you'll reach and stay in a state of ketosis.

At first glance, the keto diet could appear to be full of "junk." After all, you eat much cheese, butter, and oils. I'll admit this was the hardest thing for me to get used to, especially after years on the Paleo diet, where I stayed away from dairy completely. But what you'll find in keto is that quality matters. You want high-fat, high-quality dairy and oils, preferably grass-fed and organic (if your budget allows). The diet is still mostly grain-free and free of added sugars—just like the Paleo diet.

After a few days on keto, I not only got used to the new rules but also ended up feeling glad that so much fat (especially dairy) was not just allowed but encouraged. Do keep in mind, though, that the ketogenic diet is certainly an alternative one, so make sure to talk to your health care provider about it if you have questions, especially if you have any health issues such as heart disease or high cholesterol.

The Easiest Low-Carb Diet There Is

When I first started reading about keto, my initial thought was, There's no way I'm going to be able to do this, and I suspect it's the same for many people. I used a keto calculator to figure out all my macros, and, with my height and weight goal, I was allowed about 25 grams of carbs per day—that's the same amount of carbs as in one apple! But once you begin and get over that initial hump (a little sugar withdrawal combined with the thought, What am I supposed to eat next?), you'll find keto is very easy to stick to. This is what a typical day might look like for me in terms of meals and snacks:

- Breakfast: 2 bacon slices, Perfect Scrambled Eggs, ½ avocado

- Snack: Coconut Butter Coffee or a cup of tea with coconut oil

- Lunch: Cobb Salad

- Snack: Cheese Crisps, pork rinds, or raw veggies with Ranch Dressing.

- Dinner: Grilled steak or a cheeseburger without a bun—The Classic Juicy Lucy would be perfect—plus a side salad with Ranch Dressing, and sautéed zucchini.

- Dessert/Snack: Small handful of raspberries or a Basic Sweet Fat Bomb.

But Wait, It's Not That Easy

While I'm a big advocate of the ketogenic diet being straightforward and accessible, there's indeed a learning curve, and you have to plan and be willing to cook. I would say that planning and cooking are most certainly among the hardest parts—there are very few keto-friendly takeout options!

Luckily for you, you're reading this book, so you already know what to make and eat! Planning your meals ahead and always having snacks on hand will make your life on the ketogenic diet a lot easier and is the key to keto success. You'll also want to track everything you eat through an app such as MyFitnessPal or something similar; that way, you can see what your day looks like and begin to learn which foods work for your goals.

Real Food, Really Simple

Because keto has become such a popular diet, there are some differing opinions on what is and isn't keto, how to balance macros and best practices for generally implementing the diet into one's lifestyle in a way that's both effective and sustainable. It can take a lot of prep work to eat this way, and when so many recipes out there have numerous ingredients and long cooking times, it might seem almost impossible to come up with meals that work for you.

As noted already, there's a learning curve when it comes to keto, but other than that, the diet isn't a mystery—it's just smart eating using basic, familiar ingredients. The sooner you identify the most nutritious, keto-valuable food groups, the easier it will be for you to start eating well on a diet. Once you know what's what and get used to it all, living on the diet will come easily to you.

Take me, for example—I know that to stay in ketosis, I need to eat about 25 grams of carbs (7% of the day's allotment), 76 grams of protein (21%), and 114 grams of fat (72%) every day. After a few weeks, I learned what I needed to get from the grocery store to meal plan one week at a time so that

I could hit those numbers every day. I learned which breakfasts worked, what I should have for lunch, good ideas for dinner, and what kinds of snacks I should have between meals (if any—keto food is super filling, and you'll probably find yourself eating less frequently than you used to).

This book will help you in two key ways:

1. It's full of keto-friendly recipes that offer meal ideas and help you plan your diet in a way that's organized and effective, so you know what to buy at the grocery store and how to cook it, so it's delicious and nutritious.

2. Nutritional info is included with the recipes and variations to make calculating your macros that much easier. (When I first started, I had to log every single ingredient into MyFitnessPal to make sure my macros added up the way they were supposed to.) If you stick to the meals and snacks in this book, it should be very easy to track everything and be that much closer to reaching your goals.

Time-Sensitive, Budget-Friendly

I've said it before, and I'll say it again: If you're going to eat a special diet, you're going to have to cook. This is especially true for keto (and Paleo) diets. Because you'll be spending more time grocery shopping and cooking than you might be used to, most recipes in this book can be made in 30 minutes or fewer. If something takes longer than 30 minutes, it's probably a larger recipe or one that will last you longer than a few meals, which will save you time later in the week. You're busy; you want to spend time with your family and friends or doing the things that interest you, and spending hours in the kitchen may not be something that sounds fun.

You won't find any hard-to-come-by ingredients either, and I've kept to a minimum any recipes that include almond flour or specialty ingredients that can raise your grocery bill. I like cooking with straightforward, everyday ingredients that fit my values. I hope you'll find this helpful as you start your keto journey.

Eat This, Less Of That, And None Of Those

Keto is great because it's pretty customizable—if you don't tolerate dairy or want to stay Paleo you can just avoid cheese, heavy cream, and other dairy products, but otherwise, you could look at the diet, basically, as a low-carb, high-fat version of the Paleo diet. It's grain-free, sugar-free, and, except for dairy, generally free of most processed and packaged foods. Here's a list to get you started.

ENJOY

Avocado

Bone broth

Butter and ghee

Coconut oil

Condiments: mayonnaise, mustard, pesto, pickles, and fermented foods such as kimchi and sauerkraut

Dairy products, full-fat, such as cheese and heavy cream

Eggs

Fatty fish and seafood

Grass-fed beef

Leafy greens, including spinach and kale

Most nonstarchy vegetables, including zucchini, summer squash, cucumber, and celery

Pasture-raised lamb, pork, and poultry

Some nuts: almonds, macadamias, pecans

Water, black coffee, and tea

LIMIT

Limiting these foods will look different for every individual based on the rest of their diet—for example, someone who sweetens their morning coffee with Stevia every day is going to have fewer carbs left to also indulge in the occasional glass of dry wine or piece of dark chocolate. A lot of this also depends on whether you're actively trying to lose weight or have reached a maintenance stage of keto, where you can allow a few more carbs than you usually would. To make sure your macros are right (and to help you figure out what you have room for in your diet), stick to consistent tracking of your food intake and make sure your weight and goals are always updated in an app like MyFitnessPal or your favorite food/weight tracker.

Alcohol, to dry red and white wines or liquors (without sugary mixers)

Bacon and sausage with lots of preservatives and added sugars

Berries

Cocoa and dark chocolate

Edamame

Gluten-free soy sauce (or tamari)

Low-carb sweeteners, such as stevia

Most nuts

Nightshades (eggplant, peppers, tomatoes)

Starchy root vegetables, such as pumpkin or sweet potato

AVOID

Anything that says "low fat" or "nonfat."

Alcohol: Beer, sugary cocktails, sweet wines

Grains of all types

Milk, especially skim

Most fruit and fruit juices

Processed foods, such as almond milk and dried fruit Sweeteners

WATER MAKES IT WORK

Drinking enough water is probably one of the most important things to remember when transitioning to keto (and once you're keto-adapted). Hydrate all day. Cutting down on carbs removes extra stores of water in your body, so it's easy to get dehydrated if you don't stay on top of your water consumption. Pay attention to symptoms such as increased thirst, dry mouth, headache, dizziness, or lethargy.

I like to sip water from a big beer glass throughout the day, regularly refilling it.

Other people have a special water bottle that keeps them on top of their intake. If you're not a plain water fan, add lemon, cucumber, mint, lime, or some combination to make it more interesting. I also love sparkling water—just make sure it's a brand that doesn't add any sugar or juice, such as LaCroix.

Not only is getting enough water important for hydration, but it also helps curb cravings, keeps you from overeating, and is just generally great for your overall health.

GO-TO PANTRY ITEMS

I've found much variety in keto recipes, which is nice, but you still need a well-stocked pantry so you don't get bored after a few weeks of eating lots of the same things (when you find meals and macros that work well, it can be easy to get stuck in a rut rather than experiment all over again).

Following are the fats, herbs, oils, nuts, and spices you'll always find in my pantry and refrigerator; consider adding them to yours.

Garlic (either whole, minced, or in powder form)

Grass-fed butter

Nut kinds of butter, such as almond or peanut

Oils: Coconut, olive, and sesame

Onion (either whole, dried, or in powder form)

Sesame seeds

Tomato paste (useful for making quick sauces or adding to casseroles)

CHAPTER 14:

The Guide to Keto Diet Meal Plan

When it comes to starting with this particular diet, it is important that you create a meal plan. But the Keto Diet meal plan does involve not only planning your meals way ahead of time but also other things. Below are the things that you need to do to be successful while following the Ketogenic Diet.

Cut The Worst Carbs Out Of Your Diet: The first thing that you need to do is to do an inventory of the foods that you consume. Once you have already created an inventory, the next thing to do is to cut the worst carbs out of your diet completely. These include sweets, bread, pastries, snacks, and many others. Try Some Light Exercise: Exercising is very important if you want to push your body to ketosis faster. Exercises allow the body to use up the free glucose in your bloodstream so that you can switch on ketosis. Don't Ignore Your Macros: The dietary macronutrients for this particular diet is divided into 60% fats, 35% proteins, and 5% carbohydrates. Moreover, a dieter needs to consume no more than 2000 kcal per day and that the carbohydrates should be kept at a minimum consumption of 20 grams per day. Don't Skimp On Protein: Protein is important for muscle building, so don't skimp on them when following this diet. However, make sure that you choose the right protein choices. Ideally, you need to consume lean and organic meats sourced from grass-fed livestock. Do Not Obsess Over Your Ketone Levels: When you are still starting with the Ketogenic Diet, it is important that you don't obsess over your ketone levels. Whether your ketone levels are high or low, what matters is that you achieve ketosis.

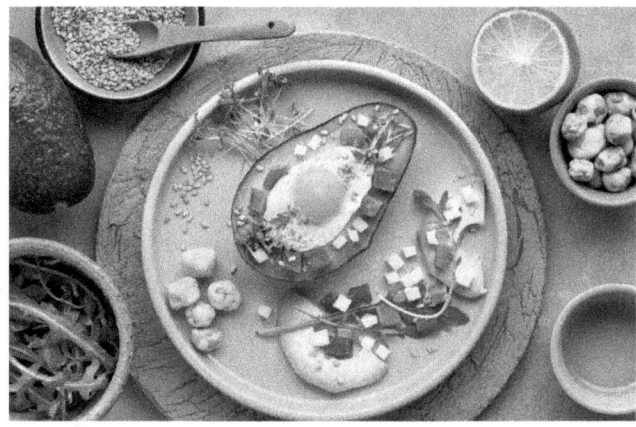

Your Body Reaction To The Meal Plan Along The Way

The increasing levels of ketone bodies in the body due to ketosis can bring about many effects on the body. The collection of the symptoms and side effects is called the Keto Flu. Below are the things that you will expect if you follow the Ketogenic Diet.

Weight Loss: The most evident reaction to following the Ketogenic Diet is weight loss within the next few days following the diet.

Thirst: Many people who follow the Ketogenic Diet feel thirstier than usual due to water loss. High levels of ketone bodies can lead to dehydration as well as electrolyte imbalance, so be sure that you drink a lot of water.

Muscle Cramps And Spasms: Because it is easy for people following the Ketogenic Diet to become dehydrated, muscle cramps and spasms may be common side effects due to electrolyte imbalance.

Headaches: Headaches can be common side effects once you switch to this diet regimen. It can happen due to the consumption of fewer carbs. However, the side effects usually last for only a few days after starting the diet.

Fatigue And Weakness: During the initial stages of the Ketogenic Diet, you might feel tired and weak than usual. This happens because the body is still adjusting after making the switch to a low carb diet.

Stomach Upset: Making any changes with your diet can increase the risk of digestive complaints. To reduce the risk, make sure that you drink plenty of liquid.

Disrupted Sleep: Disrupted sleep is a common side effect among people who switch to the Ketogenic Diet. However, this side effect usually goes away after a few weeks.

Bad Breath: Bad breath is a common side effect due to ketosis. As the ketone bodies leave the body, it produces a certain type of smell. Now, if the ketone body produced by the body is acetone, then the breath can smell fruity or sweet. However, acetopheNone and BHB can contribute to bad breath. Better Concentration: As the symptoms fade over time, most people notice that they have better concentration following the Ketogenic Diet.

Tips and FAQs

The Ketogenic Diet can help many people achieve their weight loss goals. While it encourages the consumption of fewer carb-rich food, there are other things that you can do to drive ketosis in your body. This will discuss tips and tricks to enjoy and optimize your results for this particular diet regimen.

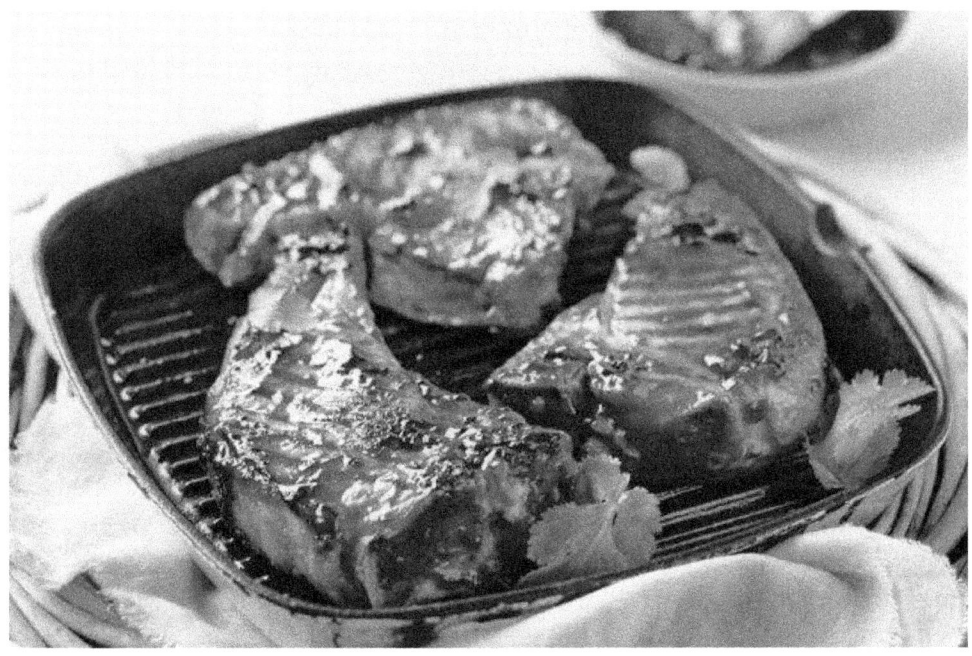

Most Common Keto Diet Mistakes You Should Know

Even if you reach your 50s, that doesn't necessarily mean that you can't make a mistake, especially when starting something new like the Ketogenic diet. Many beginners, irrespective of age, make the same mistakes when following the low-carb diet. Check out the list of the top mistakes people often make and avoid them if you want to get brilliant results from such an effective diet.

Inadequate Fluid Intake. On a keto diet, the body tries to burn more fat, and that's why it needs to be well-hydrated. Most people focus just on what they're eating and forget about what they're sipping. This mistake leads to a slower metabolism and, thus, halting weight-shedding. Besides, water is essential for nutrient circulation and flushing out toxins. So if you're going to fasten your ketosis and improve your health, try to consume 3-4 liters of water (or even more) per day.

Dairy Over-Enrichment. Remember, moderation is the key for you. Of course, you may find that dairy products are great for the Keto dieting plan. They're ideal high-fat and low-carb sources. However, don't forget that some dairy products contain sugar and overeating them can destroy your dieting plan. Due to this, you need to calculate the dairy products' calories and pay attention to their nutrition labels.

Lack of Fat. When it comes to the Keto diet, it means not just a low-carb, but also high-fat intake. At least 75% of the calories you consume should be provided from animal fats, monounsaturated fats, and olive oil. In such away, you can ensure normal hormone function and boost your metabolism.

Excess Protein Intake. We've drawn attention to the fact that if you eat too much protein, it'll cause adverse effects. Excess protein will be converted into glucose by your body, and this can ruin your dietary needs.

You were not Preparing Yourself for 'Fat Adaptation.' It can be a bit time-consuming for your body to get used to burning off fat instead of glucose for fuel. So you should prepare yourself and your body as well to experience the 'Fat Adaptation' or 'Keto Flu.' During the first week and even the second one, you may feel more fatigued, aches, and muscle cramps. That's pretty normal when your body adapts to another dietary need.

Concealment from Your doctor. Think about your age... Your doctor has the right to know about every change in your life. And especially when it comes to nutritional changes. Talk to your doctor before including Keto products in your diet plan to make sure that this's a good idea for you, and it won't harm your health.

CHAPTER 15:

What Does The Keto Diet Body Changes After 50?

We are all getting older. Of course, you are no exception. This process is inevitable, and it makes your life saturated in all aspects. When you're 50-something, you gain wisdom and life experience, you build meaningful relationships and mental strength. But don't forget that not only internal changes occur after age 50. Your body also changes, and you need to prepare for that.

Your Metabolic Rate Slows Down

When you have reached the age of 50, your body starts digesting food differently as a result of a decreased metabolic rate. Chemical reactions inside your body that are responsible for burning the calories you consume become slower. It is entirely normal and doesn't mean that you should eat less or reduce the portion sizes on your plate. This peculiarity implies that you should pay more attention to your meal plan as you age and choose the food that fits best for your nutritional needs as well as goals.

Your Muscle Power Decreases

At the old age, muscle mass and, therefore, strength reduces. Physical inactivity and an unhealthy diet are the leading causes of this negative change in a 50-something-year-old's body. But it is in your power to prevent this change.

Your Bones Become More Brittle

When it comes to the bones, you have to understand that their condition is also more likely to change after 50. Hormonal imbalance and loss of calcium and other crucial minerals in bones result in low bone density and a higher risk of injury.

Your Excess Weight Increases

Perhaps the only thing that rises with age is the figure on your scales. As you get older, you can experience disappointing changes in your body. In most cases, you notice them when looking in the mirror and weighing yourself. Extra pounds are a real problem for people who are over 50, and the most unpleasant task is getting rid of this dead weight. Well, this is one more reason why you need to focus on the Keto diet and look closely at all the benefits of this low-carb eating plan for older people.

Improved Physical and Mental Health

With aging, you might notice an energy level drop due to different environmental and biological reasons. If you want to feel happy, active, and dynamic, pay closer attention to the Keto diet. Remember, reducing your carbohydrate intake usually leads to increasing your vital forces. When you start consuming a lower number of carbs, the body has to burn more fat to fuel itself. This process causes fat synthesis and ketone production, i.e., breaking down accumulated fat for energy. In such a way, the low-carbohydrate diet can stimulate brainpower and positive changes in cognition (like improving memory and concentration).

Faster Metabolism

As already said in the older people have a slower metabolism. But thanks to the Keto diet, this problem can be solved. Excluding carb intake from your diet plan can help you to maintain healthy levels of blood sugar and, as a result, rev up your metabolism.

Weight-Shedding

It is no big secret that as a person gets older, shedding weight gets harder. People after 50 face the challenge of weight-loss for a variety of reasons (from increasing levels of stress, slower metabolic rate too rapid muscle loss). The struggle with excess weight may take a lot of time and effort for people over the age of 50. But there is a way out, and it is called the Keto diet.

This peculiar diet is highly effective for losing weight because it boosts the metabolism of fat, and the body itself starts shedding stored fat. As a bonus, people who stick to the Keto diet get a reduced appetite, which helps to prevent over-eating and, thus, quicker weight loss. Unlike many low-fat diets, the Ketogenic one doesn't recommend you to track your calories or eat less. There's no need for that! Keto usually leaves you feeling full and satisfied after a meal.

Better Sleep

At an old age, people tend to have trouble sleeping. Many people over 50 experience such sleep disorders as insomnia, sleep apnea, restless leg syndrome, and sleepwalking. People aged 50 and over should know that a long-term Ketogenic diet can have a positive impact on sleep. A significant reduction in carb intake and, at the same time, a substantial increase in fat intake create favorable conditions for a night of deeper sleep, eliminate certain sleep disturbance triggers, and make a person more energetic when the sun is up.

Protection from Age-Related Diseases

According to various scientific studies, the Keto diet can reduce the risks for specific age-related diseases, such as diabetes, different kinds of cancer, cardiovascular diseases, mental disorders, Parkinson's Disease, multiple sclerosis, and fatty liver disease.

How to Start after 50?

As you get older, it gets harder for you to make decisions. But if you want to gain more energy and stay fit in your 50s, you should try the Keto diet. Below, you'll find the complete guide for beginners.

Here are some simple steps that'll help you start the low-carb diet successfully:

Reduce Your Carb Intake to 20 Grams per Day

This is the crucial rule of the Keto diet because only if the carb levels are very-very low can your body produce ketones. However, this rule doesn't refer to fiber that can be highly effective in stimulating ketone levels.

Keep Moderate Protein Consumption

Here, 'moderate' means no less than 25 percent of calories. For example, if your weight is 70 kilos, you can eat about 100 grams of protein per day. You should know that consuming too much protein can stop ketosis because the body can turn excess protein into glucose.

Consume enough Fat

The essence of this diet is increasing fat intake. So you add enough fat to your meals to feel full. Just try not to overeat and not to eat when you don't feel hungry.

Practice Intermittent Fasting

If you skip one or two meals during the day several times a week, this can also stimulate ketosis as well as speed up weight loss.

Regulate Sleep Patterns

People over 50 should sleep 8-9 hours per night. Keep that in mind as sleep deprivation may cause slower ketosis.

Stay Active

Inserting any kind of physical activity when sticking to the Keto diet may also speed up ketosis. This is not a requirement. However, visiting a sports gym can have a positive effect not only on physical but also mental health.

The Keto diet isn't so unique and quite easy to do. However, for most older people, it can be rather challenging to adapt to it at first. According to studies, it commonly takes 21 days to make a new habit. That's why you should be patient if you want to reach your goal.

CHAPTER 16:

Basic Fitness for the Ketogenic Diet

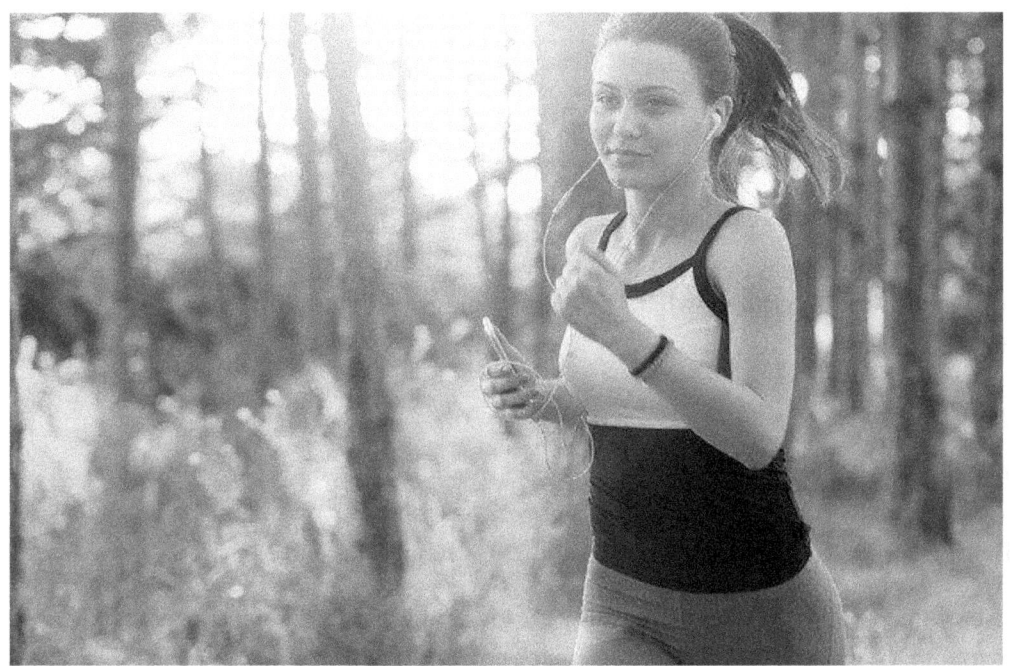

Whether you are following a Ketogenic Diet or not, exercise is almost always beneficial. As you begin to change your diet, you will experience rapid health changes already, but with exercise, you will be able to take your health to a whole new level!

As mentioned earlier, it can be slightly difficult to begin exercise routines when your body is first learning how to get into ketosis. When you are first starting, you will want to try your best to keep things light but still get your body moving. The question is, how do exercise and the Ketogenic Diet relate?

Ketogenic Diet Impact On Exercise Performance

When you first start the Ketogenic Diet, you will be restricting your carbs. As this process happens, you will be limiting the sugar access for your muscle cells. Once your muscles lack this sugar, they will begin to lose their ability to function at high intensities. For this purpose, high intensities are any activity that can last more than ten seconds.

Due to this process, any activity in the muscle that requires max effort for anywhere from ten seconds to 120 seconds requires sugar. The thing about fat and ketones is that it cannot and never will stand-in for sugar. It is after two minutes of exercise that your body knows how to shift its metabolic pathways and starts burning fat and ketones.

For this reason, you will want to avoid any extreme exercise Some popular examples include

HIIT (High-Intensity Interval Training)

Sports such as Lacrosse and Soccer

Swimming

Lifting Weights

What To Eat While Exercising On Keto

If you do plan on exercising while on a Ketogenic Diet, it is going to be vital that you get your macronutrients down. Of course, what you eat is going to depend on your goals. Are you looking to gain muscle or lose weight?

Muscle Gain

If you are looking to gain muscle on the Ketogenic Diet, you are going to want to eat more keto-friendly foods. On average, you will want to consider eating anywhere from 250-500 calories extra per day. By doing this, you will be increasing your body weight as well.

Next, most of the calories should be coming from fat. Most athletes put protein as their most important macro, but that isn't true on the Ketogenic Diet. Inf act, your protein intake should only be around one gram of protein per lean body mass that you have. On that note, is carb restriction is impairing your exercise, you may want to consider intermittent fasting.

Fat Loss

When it comes to fat loss, remember that slow loss is still a loss. As you first begin your new diet, you are going to notice weight loss without any exercise, anyway. Generally, you will want to cut down on calories anywhere between 250 and 500 calories. Weight loss comes down to calorie deficit. If you are overweight or obese, you may want to consider a higher calorie deficit.

If you still fail to lose weight after several weeks, consider lower fat intake. That seems counterproductive on the Ketogenic Diet; however, fat is still high in calories. You can still make a majority of your meal's fact-based, but enjoy them in smaller portions.

Cardio On Keto

One of the best options for beginners of the Ketogenic Diet is going to be cardio! Cardio is great for all ages because you don't have to exercise at high-intensities to gain results. As long as you are getting that heart rate up, you will be able to improve your health in some different ways.

When you are doing your cardio, you will want to try your best to maintain a moderate intensity. For this, your target heart rate should be 50-80% of your maximum heart rate. For an average 50-year old, your heart rate should be anywhere between 85 and 119 bpm.

Some of my favorite cardio exercises include:

Aerobics

Recreational Sports (with Rest Time)

Light Circuit Training

Walking

Cycling

Tips And Tricks For Maximizing Benefits

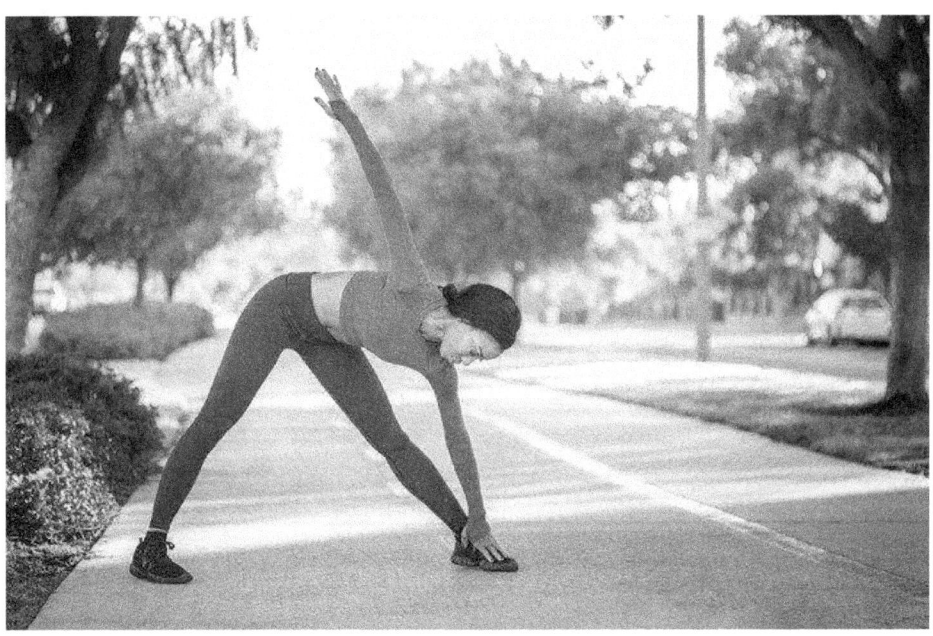

If you do plan on exercising on your diet, the good news is that there are plenty of supplements to help you get to your results quicker and more efficiently. As you pick out your supplements, be sure that they are no-carb. Below, you will find some of my favorite workout supplements.

Creatine

If you are still considering weightlifting on your new diet, you will want to look into purchasing a creatine supplement. This is safe and can enhance your phosphagen system. Generally, you will want to take about five grams a day to help you increase your power, strength, and muscle mass.

Caffeine

Caffeine is very popular among those who exercise regularly. While it can improve exercise performance, it could potentially decrease your ketone production. For this reason, you will want to consider limiting your caffeine intake, but it works when you need something at the moment.

MCT Oil

As you learned earlier, MCT is a saturated fat that is digested right away. When you need a boost of energy for endurance or cardio, you can always add some MCT oil to your meal before you exercise. Generally, anywhere between one to two tablespoons should do the trick!

CHAPTER 17:

Handling Possible Keto Reactions

Everybody is praising the special keto diet, as it gives noticeable results in the weight loss procedure. But before starting the keto diet, you should be aware of the side effects caused by it, and you can decide whether it is fine for you or not.

As the keto diet involves an extremely low carb diet and high-fat intake, it causes the metabolic state in the body called ketosis. Ketones produce because the process of ketosis burns the fats more effectively.

When you start a new way of diet, several side effects occur as the body experiences different kinds of intake and works accordingly. In the ketogenic diet, the energy switched from using glucose in carbohydrates to use the fat. This leads to a few common side effects like:

Salt Loss

In the first week of the keto diet, there is a gradual change in fluid balance in the body. As the body starts to use its stored sugar in the form of glycogen, through which the water is released into the blood and passed out from the body through urine. When the fluids pass out, the body salt also gets depleted from the body too. As in result, a person can experience excess loss of salt in the form of fluid from the body while maintaining ketosis.

To prevent the salt loss, keep hydrated all day. Water consumption is a necessity for you. Ensure that you are taking in the amount of salt in your food, as you can experience wooziness or headaches. You can also use sea salt if needed. Magnesium and potassium are very important salts. Try to take natural foods like nuts, dairy, meat, etc.

Ketosis

Ketosis is a process in which the body converts the stored fat into the energy and produces ketones as a by-product, which helps in maintaining a fast-metabolic state. This process is used to facilitate a weight loss strategy. The energy source that comes from carbohydrates is diverted, and the body starts to use body fat, resulting in fat loss.

People with diabetes experience ketosis as the body doesn't make enough insulin to process the glucose of the body. The presence of by-product, ketones in the past-out fluid – urine, indicates the amount in diabetes.

When the process of ketosis starts, a person starts to feel temporary side effects such as headaches, fatigue, brain fog, irritation, trouble sleeping, nausea, stomach-aches, dizziness, sugar intake cravings, etc.

Ketoacidosis

People, especially with diabetes, need to monitor their ketone levels with much care. Having a too high level of ketones can cause ketoacidosis in a person. The high level of ketones causes poisoning the body, causing the dangerous and severe condition, which develops rapidly. The illnesses cause a higher level of hormonal changes that start to work against insulin. Some early symptoms include abdominal pain, flushed or dry skin, confused concentration, dry mouth, urination, vomiting, nausea, etc.

Keto-flu

After some time, when you start the keto diet if you feel annoyed, experience periodic headaches, or have a hard time concentrating, then you are facing keto-flu. Although keto-flu is not an epidemic or dangerous, it is still very unpleasant to have.

Keto-flu may occur after the 3 5 days after your diet starts. Well, it is a temporary stage, and you can feel perfectly all right after the phase passes. The symptoms of keto-flu include headaches, fatigue, brain fog, dizziness, irritation from everything, high sugar cravings, lack of motivation, etc.

The reason why keto-flu occurs is that, when the body switches from high carb intake to low carb intake, the insulin level of the body lowers. As in result, ketosis occurs. It takes time for your body and brain to adopt the changes and having a new fuel.

To cure the symptoms of keto-flu, there are few steps you can take to recover from them and make your body habitual of the keto diet.

Increase in water and salt intake:

As the body salt is excreted out by the body in the process of ketosis along with water, increasing the intake can reduce your symptoms and may eliminate them for you significantly. Whenever you feel dizzy or nauseous, have a glass of water along with a half teaspoon of salt in it. This will alleviate the symptom within 15 to 30 minutes.

More fat:

Water intake and salt management can cure your symptoms, but if you want an alternative, then have more fats in your diet. There is misinformation about the fat that spreads the fatphobia among the people fighting obesity. If you are lowering your carbs and not increasing your fat consumption, you will feel hungrier, tired, and miserable.

Constipation

Constipation is another side effect of the keto diet, especially when a person diverts onto a low carb diet for the first time. The digestive system needs time to adapt to the changes and patterns of food intake. To avoid constipation, you can follow these remedies:

Water consumption:

Dehydration causes constipation. If you are having plenty of water intake, the body will absorb the water, and the dryness will not occur, which caused constipation.

Fiber intake:

You can have plenty of vegetables in your diet, which is the perfect source of fiber intake. Having a good amount of fiber intake helps the intestine work properly, which reduces the risks of constipation.

Keto Rash

Prurigo pigmentosa, known as keto rash, is another rare side effect of the keto diet, causing an inflammatory condition of the skin. Typical symptoms include redness of the skin, itchy rashes around the neck and truck, papules (red spots), rash on abdomen, and a dark brown pattern after the disappearance of spots. It is a type of dermatitis, which is more common in Asian women, according to research. Researchers cannot be entirely certain about the exact reason or cause for keto rash, but few thought it to relate to some associated conditions like Sjogren's syndrome, still are a disease and H. Pylori infection. The strong correlation between the rashes and the presence of the ketosis in the body is why it is called keto rash.

A few of the treatments include:

Carbohydrate intake:

If you think your change in diet or switching to keto diet caused you the rash, try to bring the carbohydrates back into your diet. This will help you to improve the rashes. If you do not want to compromise your keto diet, then go for more moderate low-carb options instead.

Nutritional deficiency:

The deficiency of some nutrients can also cause rashes. Deficiency of vitamin B-12, Vitamin A, and C are directly linked to acute skin conditions. While having a moderate diet, there is a possibility that your body is not getting the right amount of the minerals and vitamins that caused you the rashes. Try to have colorful fruits and vegetables in your diet to complete your deficiencies.

Skincare:

Maybe you have a sensitive skin type, which can detect the change in your body system more quickly than your fat. Take care of your skin as much as possible. Use cleansers, gentle soaps, and lukewarm water to take a bath.

Diet:

If you have a rash as a result of your keto diet, do not change your diet too quickly. Let your body accept the diet. Gradually switch to a low-carb diet with high-fat intake.

Kidney and Heart Damage

As the body becomes low in electrolytes, and the urination increases as in result, electrolytes like magnesium, sodium, and potassium levels decrease. This can make you prone to acute injury of the kidney in some cases. Dehydration may lead to serious results like kidney stones, kidney injury, or light-headedness. Also, for a normal beating of the heart, electrolytes are necessary. If proper diet and precautions are not taken, then a person would face some serious problems as well.

Cramps in Legs

Cramps in legs are common when you switch to a low-carb diet. It is a minor issue, but painful. It is mainly caused by the loss of minerals from the body, especially magnesium. There are simple ways to avoid these legs cramps:

Drink water and maintain your salt intake

Use a magnesium supplement if needed

Bad Breath

While following a strict keto diet, some people observed the smell from their breath, like nail polish remover or acetone. The smell the ketone is producing in the result of ketone formation in the body, which is, in fact, a sign that your body is burning much fat and producing ketones to fuel your organs. If you are sweating a lot, this can be turned into your body odor.

To avoid the bad breath, observe proper oral hygiene along with a good intake of water, breath freshener, etc.

Energy Loss

Another misconception regarding keto diet is that glucose represents the energy level of the body. To maintain an appropriate level of energy is way more challenging while having a standard diet, as it fluctuates according to the food intake and blood sugar level.

You may feel your energy level is low at the beginning of your diet when your body is adopting the phase, but it is temporary and will be fine after a week or two, so do not worry.

CHAPTER 18:

Benefits of Following Keto Diet for Women Over 50

The Keto diet has been proven to have many benefits for people over 50. Here are some of the best.

Strengthens bones

When people get older, their bones weaken. At 50, your bones are likely not as strong as they used to be. However, you can keep them in really good condition. Consuming milk to get calcium cannot do enough to strengthen your bones. What you can do is to make use of the Keto diet as it is low in toxins. Toxins negatively affect the absorption of nutrients, and so with this, your bones can take in all they need.

Eradicates inflammation

Few things are worse than the pain from an inflamed joint or muscle. Arthritis, for instance, can be extremely difficult to bear. When you follow the ketosis diet, the production of cytokines will be reduced. Cytokines cause inflammation, and therefore, their eradication will reduce it.

It eradicates nutrients deficiency

Keto focuses on consuming exactly what you need. If you use a great Keto plan, your body will lack no nutrients and will not suffer any deficiency.

Reduced hunger

The reason we find it difficult to stick to diets is hunger. It doesn't matter your age; diets do not become easier. We may have a mental picture of the healthy body we want. We may even have clear visuals of the kind of life we want to lead once free from unhealthy living, but none of that matters when hunger enters the scene. However, the Keto diet is a diet that combats this problem. The Keto diet focuses on consuming plenty of proteins. Proteins are filling and do not let you feel hungry too easily. Besides, when your carb levels are reduced, your appetite takes a hit. It is a win-win situation.

Weight loss

Keto not only burns fat, but it also reduces that craving for food. Combined, these are two great ways to lose weight. It is one of the diets that has proven to help the most when it comes to weight loss. The Keto diet has been proven to be one of the best ways to burn stubborn belly fat while keeping yourself revitalized and healthy.

Reduces blood sugar and insulin

After 50, monitoring blood sugar can be a real struggle. Cutting down on carbs drastically reduces both insulin levels and blood sugar levels. This means that the Keto diet will benefit millions as many people struggle with insulin complications and high blood sugar levels. It has been proven to help as when some people embark on Keto, and they cut up to half of the carbs they consume. It's a treasure for those with diabetes and insulin resistance. A study was carried out on people with type 2 diabetes. After cutting down on carbs, within six months, 95 percent of people were able to reduce or stop using their glucose-lowering medication.

Lower levels of triglycerides

Many people do not know what triglycerides are. Triglycerides are molecules of fat in your blood. They are known to circulate the bloodstream and can be very dangerous. High levels of triglycerides can cause heart failures and heart diseases. However, Keto is known to reduce these levels.

Reduces acne

Although acne is mostly suffered by those who are young, there are cases of people above 50 having it. Moreover, Keto is not only for persons after 50. Acne is not only caused by blocked pores. There are quite some things proven to cause it. One of these things is your blood sugar. When you consume processed and refined carbs, it affects gut bacteria and results in the fluctuation of blood sugar levels. When the gut bacteria and sugar levels are affected, the skin suffers. However, when you embark on the Keto diet, you cut off on carbs intake, which means that in the very first place, your gut bacteria will not be affected, thereby cutting off that avenue to develop.

Increases HDL levels

HDL refers to high-density lipoprotein. When your HDL levels are compared to your LDL levels and are not found low, your risk of developing heart disease is lowered. This is great for persons over 50 as heart diseases suddenly become more probable. Eating fats and reducing your intake of carbohydrates is one of the most certain ways to increase your high-density lipoprotein levels.

Reduces LDL levels

High levels of LDL can be very problematic when you attain 50. This is because LDL refers to bad cholesterol. People with high levels of this cholesterol are more likely to get heart attacks. When you reduce the number of carbs you consume, you will increase the size of bad LDL particles. However, this will result in the reduction of the total LDL particles as they would have increased in size. Smaller LDL particles have been linked to heart diseases, while larger ones have been proven to have lower risks attached.

May help combat cancer

I termed this under 'may' because research on this is not as extensive and conclusive as we would like it to be. However, there is proof of supporting it. Firstly, it helps reduce the levels of blood sugar, which in turn reduces insulin complications, which in turn reduces the risk of developing cancers related to insulin levels. Besides, Keto places more oxidative stress on cancer cells than on normal cells, thereby making it great for chemotherapy. The risk of developing cancer after fifty is still existent, and so, Keto is a lifesaver.

May lower blood pressure

High blood pressure plagues adults much more than it does young ones. Once you attain 50, you must monitor your blood pressure rates. Reduction in the intake of carbohydrates is a proven way to lower your blood pressure. When you cut down on your carbs and lower your blood sugar levels, you greatly reduce your chances of getting some other diseases.

Combats metabolic syndrome

As you grow older, you may find that you struggle to control your blood sugar level. Metabolic syndrome is another condition that has been proven to influence diabetes and heart disease development. The symptoms associated with metabolic syndrome include but are not limited to high triglycerides, obesity, high blood sugar level, and low levels of high-density lipoprotein cholesterol.

However, you will find that reducing your level of carbohydrate intake greatly affects this. You will improve your health and majorly attack all the above-listed symptoms. Keto diet helps to fight against metabolic syndrome, which is a big win.

Great for the heart

People over the age of 50 have been proven to have more chances of developing heart diseases. Keto diet has been proven to be great for the heart. As it increases good cholesterol levels and reduces the levels of bad cholesterol, you will find that partaking in the Keto diet proves extremely beneficial for your health.

May reduce seizure risks

When you change your intake levels, the combination of protein, fat, and carbs, as we explained before, your body will go into ketosis. Ketosis has been proven to reduce seizure levels in people who have epilepsy. When they do not respond to treatment, the ketosis treatment is used. This has been done for decades.

Combats brain disorders

Keto doesn't end there, and it also combats Alzheimer's and Parkinson's disease. Some parts of your brain can only burn glucose, and so, your body needs it. If you do not consume carbs, your lover will make use of protein to produce glucose. Your brain can also burn ketones. Ketones are formed when your carb level is very low. With this, the ketogenic diet has been used f r plenty of years to treat epilepsy in children who aren't responding to drugs. For adults, it can work the same magic as it is now being linked to treating Alzheimer's and Parkinson's disease

Conclusion

Well health food enthusiasts, that's it! You now have everything you need to embark on your nourishing. These recipes are just the beginning of your wellness journey, and there are no limits to the endless possibilities you can whip up with your Ketogenic diet!

By now, you've probably learned that you are designed to help you make far more than just homestyle baked beans like your grandma's pressure cooker. From healthy soups and appetizers to main dishes and desserts, you were designed to tackle it all! The best part? It is every chef's best friend since it is made of stainless steel that intentionally cuts out harmful chemicals, leaving only the delicious flavors of your wholesome ingredients.

Whether you are a seasoned Ketogenic eater or you are trying out this health-conscious diet for the first time, you now hold a complete guide to mastering the art of the Ketogenic Diet in a fraction of the time. Before you head out to the farmer's market and start chopping up veggies, we want to share some of our favorite tips and tricks for getting the most out of your and taking full advantage of the amazing new diet you've just started!

Unlike those fad diets you've seen advertised on TV, the Ketogenic Diet was created with busy people in mind. Whether you're grabbing a quick bite in between meetings, enjoying a healthy snack while shuffling your kids back and forth from soccer practice, or just trying to fit in a little home-style cooking into your routine, the Ketogenic Diet was designed to accommodate even the most hectic of schedules. So, how you may ask?

Well, for starters, there is no need for pre-portioned or frozen meals like other diets on the market. Sure, it's easy to eat well when you're confined to the contents of your freezer, but that leaves most of us hanging whenever we venture beyond the homestead. After all, can you schlep those packaged meals with on-the-go when your miles away from a microwave? We didn't think so!

Since the Ketogenic Diet promotes weight loss through your body's natural process of breaking down fats, you won't start craving those quick pick-me-ups that become somewhat of a survival tool with other diets. Sticking to the Ketogenic Diet creates a healthy lifestyle (not just a fad eating trend) and can re-program your body to crave nourishing, wholesome ingredients instead of quick-processing sugars or carbohydrates.

When you learn to love organic and healthy foods like those found in the Ketogenic Diet, you can learn to choose these foods when you're out and about as well! Whether you're meeting your girlfriends for appetizers after work or picking up a quick bite during your lunch break, you'll be surprised how many healthy options are out there when you start looking!

Want to take your newfound love of the Ketogenic Diet with you on-the-go? Well, you've come to the right place because that brings us to our next trip.

Ask any fitness buff about their secret to staying ripped, and we bet that they will all answer with the same sound advice: meal prepping. The key to sticking with a diet and transforming eating habits into an oops-proof lifestyle is simple: you need access to hearty, wholesome foods 24/7!

This is where you truly come in handy, fellow chefs! By far, one of the biggest perks cooking is the ability to prepare delicious meals in bulk without wasting hours upon hours in the kitchen. How does this fit with your new diet? Put it this way, there are no excuses for skipping on Ketogenic eating when you can bring your latest creations with you to work, the neighborhood potluck, or anywhere else your busy life may take you!

Ready to get started? Check out our tried and true guide to meal prepping so you can enjoy the benefits of the Ketogenic Diet anytime, anywhere!

Food Storage. You have your cookbook, organic ingredients, now what? Well, you're going to need a place to store all of that delicious food and containers to help you bring everything with you on-the-go. We recommend adding the following to your Ketogenic arsenal:

Leak-proof food storage containers in a variety of sizes (preferably glass to avoid those harmful chemicals found in plastic!);

Reusable storage bags; and

Eco-friendly food storage wraps (these are usually made of a cloth treated in beeswax and can be reused over and over again!).

Prep Station. Make room for at least one week's worth of meals by clearing off a little space on your kitchen counter, coffee table; you name it! You won't need a ton of space, just enough to line your containers up in a neat little row (or two!) so you can prep like a well-oiled machine.

A Little Time. This is our favorite part! No need to carve out an entire chunk of your day (or even a few hours), but you will want to set aside a designated time each week that is dedicated to food prep. We recommend taking advantage of your Sunday morning or afternoon; in no time at all, this will become one of your favorite weekly rituals!

A Fun Lunch Bag or Tote! Pick a color, pattern, and style that you love to pack everything in each day. The more you love it, the more likely you are to bring your Ketogenic meals with you (and the less likely you are to walk out of the house realizing you forgot your lunch on the counter…again…for the third time this week!).

Another thing we love about the Ketogenic Diet? It's perfect for the whole family! No matter how many people you have in your tribe, this healthy lifestyle is for everyone. After all, a family that eats together stays together!

Do you have little ones or picky eaters? No problem! Most of the recipes in this cookbook are healthy adaptations of the go-to meals your family already knows and loves. In fact, by substituting just a few ingredients, you may just fool those picky eaters into going carb-free without even knowing it.

Another bonus of bringing the whole family in on the Ketogenic fun? Support! Accountability and support are some of the most important factors in the success of a new healthy lifestyle, and having your family's seal of approval will make your success that much was easier to attain. When you're all in on the fun, you won't have to worry about being tempted by one person's love of fried chicken or fast food burgers, and you will have the bonus of creating a healthy, sustainable lifestyle for your entire family for years to come.

Ketogenic eating is one of the fastest-growing diets in the world, and it's easy to understand why. From weight loss to increased energy and every health benefit in between, it's no wonder that this instinctual diet is taking the world by storm. Well, just like the Ketogenic Diet has become an overnight sensation. Together, these two make one mean, green, wellness machine, and are your ticket to the healthy lifestyle you've always wanted.

Want to make the most of the recipes in this cookbook? Shop organic, locally-grown ingredients from your neighborhood farmer's market or small grocer! These ingredients are pesticide-free and typically come from the freshest farms around, so your recipes will always taste their very best! A bonus? Shopping locally supports the farmers in your community while reducing environmental harms and promoting long-lasting sustainability. Happy Cooking!

CPSIA information can be obtained
at www.ICGtesting.com
Printed in the USA
LVHW101912181020
669109LV00008B/181